THE NO COAT MEDICINE

THE NO COAT MEDICINE

A guide for living a long and healthy life

Maria Sulindro-Ma, MD. ABAAM

Xulon Press Elite

Xulon Press Elite
2301 Lucien Way #415
Maitland, FL 32751
407.339.4217
www.xulonpress.com

© 2019 by Maria Sulindro-Ma, MD. ABAAM

All rights reserved solely by the author. The author guarantees all contents are original and do not infringe upon the legal rights of any other person or work. No part of this book may be reproduced in any form without the permission of the author. The views expressed in this book are not necessarily those of the publisher.

Unless otherwise indicated, Scripture quotations taken from the King James Version (KJV) – *public domain*.

Printed in the United States of America.

Edited by Xulon Press.

Information presented in this book is intended for educational purposes only and not for individual medical advice.

Illustrations by Stacey Sugiono
Research by Oliver Sugiono

Location: Aesthetic and Anti-Aging Medicine
890 S. Arroyo Parkway
Pasadena, CA 91107

626–403–9000 Fax: 626–237–5577
E-mail: AskDrMaria@MariaMD.com
Website: www.MariaMD.com

AskDrMaria@MariaMD.com
Website: www.MariaMD.com

AskDrMaria@gmail.com

ISBN-13: 9781498454650

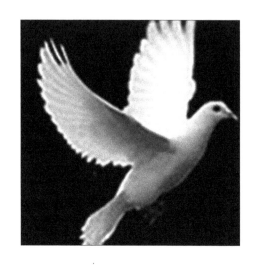

The Highest Good

To attain the highest good
Of true man and womanhood,
Simply do
Your honest best.
God with joy
Will do the rest.

—James Whitcomb Riley

TABLE OF CONTENTS

Preface ix
Forward from Dr. Ronald Klatz xi
Forward from Dr. Mark Houston xiii
The title xv
Disclaimer xvii
Dedication xix

PART ONE

1. The Introduction of Healthy Aging 3
2. The Genesis of Healthy Aging 23
3. The History of Medicine 31
4. The Wisdom of Health 35
5. The Prophetic Health 39

PART TWO

6. Introduction — Integrative Medicine:
   Journey in Healthy Aging 47
7. The Pillars 56
   Pillar I: Detoxification 68
   Pillar II: Diet & Nutrition 89
   Pillar III: Exercise and Activity 130
   Pillar IV: Stress Reduction 137
   Pillar V: Hormone Balancing 147
   Pillar VI: Cell Regeneration 176
   Pillar VII Early Detection of Diseases 180

8. The Practice and the Programs 196
9. The Results and Testimonials. 206

APPENDIX

Doctor's Contact and Information 240
Resources: Medical Organizations 243
Biological Dentist Organizations 246
Research Organizations. 246
Laboratories 247
Compounding Pharmacies. 251

BIBLIOGRAPHY and REFERENCES 255

Meet the Author 265

Preface

Have you ever asked your doctor what caused you to be sick? Often they will say, "We do not know why you are sick, but take these pills and you will feel better."

I believe asking what is the cause of your being sick is a very important question. I believe an integrative approach can reveal the answer to the cause of the symptoms that you have. While treating the symptoms, we, the integrative physicians, will show the patients that we need to correct the underlying causes. Sometimes we treat the patient to prevent sickness, using the latest in medical science. Sometimes a homeopathic approach can be tried when current technology is exhausted or does not provide a solution.

"Prolonging life is not the goal. Prolonging health is the goal." Hat good is long life if it means hobbeling around in a convalescent home out of your mind ? . If you prolong health, you will naturally prolong life. Prolonging health naturally prolongs good looks and your zest for life or vitality. You can improve your beauty on the outside to look younger, but don't forget, real youth starts within. To remain young and healthy is an investment in yourself and requires discipline. Your outer appearance will reflect your inner health.

We will supply the education about being healthy, and you will supply the discipline to follow through on our advice. Soon your friends will want to know your secret.

Foreword

DR. MARIA SULINDRO, A MEMBER OF THE AMERICAN Academy of Anti-Aging Medicine, has put together an up to date resourse, which easily explains the new modalities and therapies of Anti-Aging Medicine for the public. From Vitamins to exercise, colonics to hormones, hyperbaric oxygen to meditation. It is a readable and understandable text that will educate and inspire the reader to choose wisely from the many different modalities now available to slow aging related diseases.

From:
Dr. Ronald Klatz, MD,DO
Co-founder/President of the American Academy of Anti Aging Medicine.
http://www.worldhealth.net/pages/dr_ronald_klatz_resume/
http://www.youtube.com/watch?v=Hrhx21Tq4yU

The American Academy of Anti Aging Medicine, the A4M is headquatered in Boca Raton Florida. The A4M established in 1991 and now represents over 20.000 physician members in 120 countries.

The A4M provides continuing education to Physicians as well as Specialized training programs and a Board Certification
More information can be found at www.Worldhealth.net

Foreword

DR SULINDRO HAS PROVIDED A REALISTIC AND SIMPLE roadmap for all of us to achieve better health in her new book: THE NO COAT MEDICINE. Over 80 percent of disease can be prevented by following the program outlined in this book. Personal education and responsibility for one's health is explained in simple and understandable language to allow you to accept your mission to be accountable for your spiritual, mental and physical health and longevity. Her life story and her heart are poured out in this book. If you are ready for you to begin your journey, then read it and do it. That which lies before you, is truly amazing.

From:
Mark Houston MD, MS, MSc, FACP, FAHA, FACN, FASH, ABAARM
Associate Clinical Professor
of Medicine
Vanderbilt University Medical School
Director, Hypertension Institute and
Vascular Biology
Medical Director of Division of
Human Nutrition
Saint Thomas Medical Group, Saint
Thomas Hospital
Nashville, Tennessee

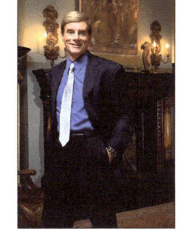

Author of What Your Doctor May Not Tell You About Hypertension, What Your Doctor May Not Tell You About Heart Disease, and Nutritional Strategies in Cardiovascular Medicine.

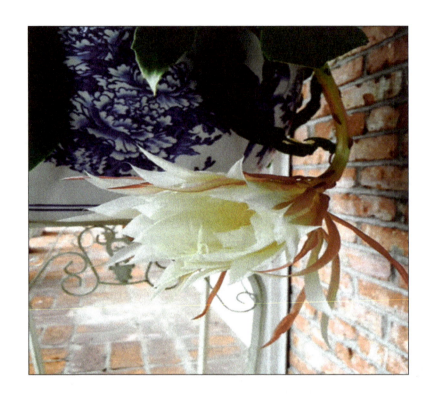

"Never be discouraged
When failures come to light-
Just use them for stepping stones
And make a stronger fight.

-Loreta Inman-

Staying healthy and feel young is the goal.

About the Title:
THE NO COAT MEDICINE

The coat stands for the doctor's coat. I was trained in Physical Medicine and Rehabilitation. I also was curious at first that the patients in the Rehabilitation wards were not required to use the hospital gowns. The hospital gown reinforces to the patient "that I am sick" not ready to be fully functional. The hospital gown says "I am a patient" not a person with questions and in control of my health.

What about the physicians? Well when we were in the hospital, we all wore the white coat. The white coat is to differentiate us from others. On our right chest area, we had our name and our title.

In contrast however, when we rotated to the private office of Rehabilitation specialist, none of the doctors wear a WHITE COAT. Here in rehab the patients also shed the hospital gown because they are preparing to go back to their real lives. They are not just patients they are co-workers with the doctors in their return to full health. This is what I feel is what Integrative medicine is all about.

We are getting healthy and happy together.

"The white coat syndrome" Implies that when the patient goes to the hospital or the doctor's office, they feel anxious and uneasy. When you check their vital signs, their blood pressure can go up, or they sometimes have sweaty, hands.

Personally I am an artist. I like everything beautiful. Nothing is beautiful about most hospitals and White Coats.

Some of my patients come for their annual evaluation so they can pass to continue being a pilot. They tell me that if I they had to go and see a White Coat doctor, they may not pass with their vital signs. So each time they come to me, I want to make sure I find something to make them calm for their physical examination.

The NO COAT seems to fit this program of integrative medicine. I am not surprised that many of the integrative medicine doctors like to wear just their casual outfit with no white coat. I hope this helps people who are wondering why the book is named NO COAT medicine.

Disclaimer

THIS BOOK IS WRITTEN AS EDUCATIONAL MATERIAL for the readers who are mainly nonmedical professionals. The words are selected so that laymen can understand, not just medical professionals. It is definitely not meant to replace medical advice or care from a primary physician or other specialist who only practices conventional or traditional medicine. The author has spent much time and has selected a good deal of information from other references, such as published scientific papers and documents. She also has four decades of clinical experience in a private setting, using a comprehensive Integrative Medicine approach. Much of the content in this book is a result of the clinical improvement of the author's patients.

All the recommendations are used for general guidelines. Adjustments should be made with consultation with one's own primary care doctors.

The author has no financial ties to any manufacturing company or laboratory at this moment; she works and earns her salary from her private practice. She allows medical students of an established conventional university to rotate through her practice without charge.

The compounded or personalized products she recommends are used for patients to get better results. They are all based on long years of clinical experience. The author is not responsible for failure to improve in the reader's health, nor is she liable for any adverse effects from using suggested products in this book. Readers should directly consult their own physician or seek direct consultation from the author at her office for any new medication, nutrition, detoxification program, or health regimen mentioned here.

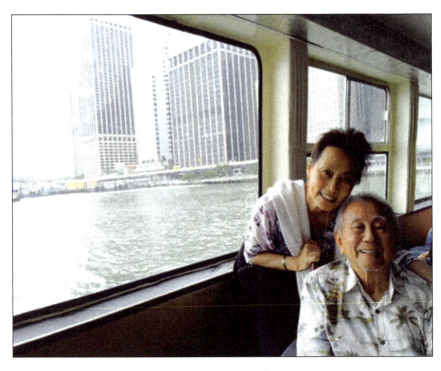

The Loving Thing

The child in me that often wished
To wipe His brow and help Him up
Each time He fell
Now knows that wish is granted us
Each time we do for any man
The loving thing.

-Edward A. Gloeggler-

Dedication

To all my friends and mentors, Herman my husband and three beautiful children, brothers and sisters, and especially my loving father, Sulindro-Ma (born in 1928). At eighty-eight years young, he is smart, full of enthusiasm, and enjoying a long active life, a living example of love, leadership, and happiness.

To all my patients, who have given me the reward of seeing them come back to me healthy and happy. They pushed me to finish this introductory book to the new field of Integrative Medicine. The American Board of Physicians Specialists has recently recognized this field officially.

To my special friend pastor Don Bennett, who helped to proofread this book. Without him, this would still be on my things-to-do list.

To my late mother who was so strong, beautiful, and smart and loved her God and family with her whole heart. She, who taught me much, said this: "You earn from the community and you need to give back to the community." She raised all her children to trust in God and believe in the family as a unit.

Last, but not least, I dedicate this book to my Creator and Provider, who gave me the "discerning spirit" and open-mindedness to pioneer this route thirty years ago. I follow this path to help more people in the world and myself to attain a long and healthy life.

Part One

Chapter 1

INTRODUCTION OF HEALTHY AGING

As a practicing clinician for almost Thirty eight years, I have been blessed to see the differences between my conventional training that was good from my holistic training. The conventional training fell short in years of real human application. I was trained as a medical doctor and turned to traditional specialties when my biological sibling had a surprising stroke at the age of thirty. We were perplexed. How could that happen?

After spending so much money to find the real cause, we could not find why we had a stroke, and I came to the conclusion that he had a "stress and acute vasoconstriction of the arteries." It was not until ten years later, a good friend and well-respected doctor sent me an e-mail from France and told me that I should look into highly sensitive C-Reactive protein (Hs-CRP). That was in 1984 when this "inflammatory marker" was not routinely checked in the United States. I called around and found a lab that was willing to do it for $1,640 and was not covered then by any insurance. The current cost is only $35, and it is now fully covered by most insurance.

Sure enough, that was the only positive evidence and possible explanation why he had a stroke. Today, even the patients understand and request that their inflammatory markers be tested. They request not only one marker but many of them. They ask for markers to be tested for cardiovascular, metabolic, and progressive chronic diseases like cancer. We managed to reduce the markers for my brother and, thank God, that has changed his condition. He has recovered with special care and of course with his own big lifestyle adjustments. He has not had any major health issues since then. He is now sixty-two years young, thirty-two years since his stroke.

This experience brought me to understand how people can be so different after a major health problem, especially with cardiovascular disease. One can became a different person, with changes in personality, emotion, and way of thinking. They find they are unable to do many previous tasks. The family members suffer as well, due to these changes.

Since then, in my opinion, physical age does not mean anything. It is how we live, adopting a healthy lifestyle, that is the key element and "secret" to recovery. It will not be a secret any more as many of you will learn as you follow the series of books I intend to write for general education. My mother taught me to be dedicated to the community we live in.

After more than thirty years of practicing as an Integrative Medicine clinician and continuous medical education in related issues or topics, I began to realize that we are entering a phase of "evolution." Some I might attribute this to communication technology in media or the Internet, it is very clear to me that a normal person would readily choose to go this holistic way where they do not have to worry about any side effects. People are demanding better care. That is the real cause of the evolution. This feeling of good health due to healthy living and holistic care, of course, results in longer biological age. This holistic style of living seems to be more popular now than thirty years ago. People come to understand that it is not just looking young and pretty or handsome that is most enjoyable, but feeling young and being healthy is the most important.

There is a saying that "money cannot buy health." I am not sure this applies in my field because to stay healthy now, requires an investment in our body. Any investment either in time or money, is going to be required. People who start this anti-aging lifestyle from birth are going to be the wealthiest people. This can start when a child is in the womb. You as parents can affect your baby if you stay healthy during the pregnancy.

When I was in high school (1968) I never thought of "healthy food." My mother started us out to be a little choosy. She taught us to remember to eat three times a day, eat my morning milk and eggs, and also not go to sleep or exercise right after meals. In my office, we had never had the idea that gluten could be dangerous. Our food and our environment have now become one of the hottest topics in conversation and regulation, such as no more smoking in public places because secondary smoke can affect us more than the smokers. People are avoiding MSG in their food. Now they have hundreds of kinds of water filtration systems to distill water to alkaline from acidic. People are looking for organic and gluten free food every where.

Sugar-free food and many types of sweeteners are available for public use. But the public knows that even if they are in this revolution of health, the medical professions are often the last and most reluctant to change. Why? When doctors have learned theories and practice in the best medical schools money can buy, they sometimes are reluctant or unwilling to change. Change is often painful. Integrative Medicine has moved very slowly for thirty years, and it may take another thirty years for the rest of the professional medical doctors to accept it for their own health and then for their patients.

That is why the life span of a doctor is lower than the average age of the general population, especially those who have strange hours (Ob-Gyns, Surgeons, and Anesthesiologists) at hospitals and those who deal with infectious diseases. Not many physicians do what they tell their patients to do. For example, I know a cardiologist who was shocked to find out that his triglyceride level was through the roof (1640), and he was probably in pancreatic shock and metabolic disease syndrome (previously called Syndrome X) at that time.

At the urging of an Integrative and Holistic Medicine doctor, instead of just taking the drugs stamped in his prescription pad, he decided to regularly take soluble fibers and supplements. After a few weeks, he was curious and checked his levels again, and to his relief he found out that his triglyceride levels had drastically lowered by 50 percent. In one month his triglycerides were regulated by diet and lifestyle changes. The next month, he resigned from his position in a prestigious medical school in Los Angeles (UCLA) and lives a healthier life, promoting diet and nutrition instead. This sudden change in a physician, who was near death, came about by experiencing a dramatic change in his condition through fiber and supplements.

Therefore, current opinions change because they have seen the worst happen when they do not change. There were people who lived in the 1800s who had this idea of living healthy already, such as Dr. Hoxey, but they were persecuted and often jailed or driven into another country. I can name a few who had those experiences while I was learning Integrative Medicine and many more who expressed their opinion and were found dead a short time after.

In the year 1776, the average age was only thirty-five years. But after 300 years, the average age now is sixty-eight, and the prediction is that by 2020, the population of people over sixty-five years old will be the largest. By 2050, 30 percent of the people on this earth will be over sixty-five. We all know that women live longer. If you are between the ages of forty and seventy and live a healthy life, you might live to eighty-five or one hundred or even older.

I have just seen a man in my office recently who is sixty-five years old and came in with stage 3 cancer. His parents lived to 100 and 106 years of age and died of old age because the father felt lonely after the mother passed away. They bore ten children and did not have any major diseases. I was impressed and am now checking why he has cancer at this young age compared to his parents. Could a toxic environment have caused his illness because he worked for twenty years as a valet parking person? The toxic inhalants from the gas and fumes would affect his immune system and cause cancer cells to actively grow and mutate. Plus, his parents lived in a rural environment and ate vegetables out of the garden, no doubt. In the city, he is exposed to high electrical currents that are now manifested through cell phones, cell phone towers, and cordless phones and even computers, microwaves, and big-screen televisions, which were not available in his parents' lives.

High-tech "gene therapy" or decoding of the genes will help, but I believe in the next few years people will pursue a long and healthy life by reading this kind of book and taking charge of their health. Suppose we live longer. That is still not our purpose. The purpose is how to live an active life and not spend time in hospitals being treated with antiquated treatments that do not support our immune systems. This vicious cycle will take its toll on you when you live with drugs as the answer to all your ailments. The health system we have today in the United States will eventually bankrupt our country. I would like to see the majority of the population live longer with healthy lives and those who are unfortunately ill as the minority of the population.

Who is going to support these ideas? As predicted thirty years ago, increasingly large numbers of people are drawn to these kinds of life-changing concepts, and we see doctors who try to treat the whole person and not just their symptoms. This has taken dedication and sacrifice from physicians for the past thirty years because no big pharmaceutical company would help to fund the studies of supplements that are not able to be patented and where profit is not high. Likewise no financial institution, such as health insurance companies, would cover this kind of medicine should the patient need supplements for their nutrition. I believe we are about to see major changes in all kinds of definitions.

Health insurance today should be called hospital insurance. We should have real health insurance where our health is the focus and not the named diseases. The "meaning of cure" in cancer might be redefined. As we know, those who are not subjected and bombarded by toxic drugs are going to survive longer if their immune systems are built up. The definition of health facilities should be changed to Urgent Care for Acute Symptoms or Chronic Symptoms. However, what we really need are cause-based treatment clinics where we look for the cause of the illness and treat that rather than just the symptoms.

Some of my patients were shocked initially when they had to take several pills (food supplements) that look like drugs on a daily basis. However, when they were tested or reevaluated again, they were usually pleasantly surprised. Some quit the program due to the biggest issue now—they run out of money. But many of them stay because the results of our treatments give them better health. They are now educated and willing to change their agenda in their lives to avoid the problems and to prevent these health issues from reoccurring.

Therefore this kind of medicine can be called also anti-aging medicine (A4M), preventive medicine, functional medicine (IFIM), age management medicine (AMM), "advancement in medicine" (ACAM.ORG), regeneration medicine (ABRM), metabolic medicine, alternative medicine, and so forth. There are too many to name. Many have their own style and ideas that they have found valuable to share. However the American Board of Physician Specialty (ABPS) has decided to call these protocols of evidence-based medicine "Integrative Medicine." Their criteria fall into the category of fellowship programs for an extra two years of formal education after the residency program. This is now being offered in some medical institutions.

The Americans hopefully will enjoy this kind of treatment very soon and not just what can be accomplished with drugs or old technology. The challenge is that sometimes your genes might be mutated already during their formation. Thanks to new technology, some supplements often compensate for even this weakness. With geriatric medicine (which is not the same), they have to learn how to minimize dosage of the drugs for the elderly. We try not to use drugs but will decide to use drugs if it is absolutely necessary and only for as short a time as possible. Now there is a conflict here because many doctors will speak condescendingly about this kind of medicine until they become patients themselves. Then suddenly, doctors who are prescribing toxic care do not want to take their own prescriptions.

Many patients still use conventional doctors because they have been well established for 300 years in the United States. Or in some cases they like their doctor and are convinced they are their friend. Of course, conventional medicine doctors are their friends and are well meaning, but that does not mean we should die for them.

Due to rapid changes in holistic medicine, many patients are adopting Integrative Medicine, which we provide. To a certain degree, self-practice without professional help or supervision will harm the patients if they are suffering from a progressive disease such as cancer, Parkinson's or Parkinsonism, Alzheimer's, Chronic Fatigue syndrome, Fibromyalgia, Migraine, and many others. If one suffers such an affliction, one needs to seek out the best specialist in that area and not try to self-medicate.

My own journey of Integrative Medicine started early in my career. My transformation took place when I already was a practicing doctor at twenty-five years of age. By age twenty-seven, I was convinced that some things are not all useful in conventional medicine. Of course, the majority of conventional treatments are well received by the health insurance companies. But that is if you solely depend on the third-party payer to take care of your health as many people do in this country. Unlike in Asia, people pay out of pocket when they go to see their doctors; therefore Integrative Medicine is widely accepted there and in many socialized countries. In the long run, Integrative Medicine's cost is much lower as people are avoiding all the side effects that can accumulate while taking drugs approved by the FDA (Food Drugs Administration). Only the approved drugs have claimed side effects. Those drugs not approved by FDA, but are "regulated by the FDA," are the ones that have no side effects; thus approval is not required.

Since I was fourteen years old, while studying, I often felt suddenly dizzy and then fainted. In our family, a "punishment" for not following house rules was to stand in a corner for a long time in one spot. I could not tolerate this very long. I was in a junior high school in Singapore then. I also experienced cold sweats after lack of sleep or severe muscle cramps after stretching or after a swimming competition where extra effort was required. These kinds of unpleasant experiences became worse when I attended college and medical school. Often I could not finish brushing my teeth in the morning without getting dizzy. As it continued to become worse, my arms and leg muscles would twitch, my skin would become rough, and my face would break out in pimples.

All of the above began at around sixteen years of age. In 1973, I entered a medical school program where studying was mandatory. My parents thought I was lazy because all my friends were studying past midnight, and I was found sleeping in the guest room after 7:00 p.m. In classes where slide shows were given and lights were dimmed, I would fall asleep. I could not open my eyes even if I heard the teacher. He would use a flashlight to shine into my closed eyes and try to wake me up. My friends wondered what was wrong. My struggle peaked when I could not go in the morning to reach my campus. My parents were panicky, and I was hospitalized.

An EMG test was done on my muscles, and they found muscle fatigue but no other neurological findings. Miraculously, I survived the lengthy clinical rotations. I completed my formal conventional medical school training. Long story short, I arrived in the United States and pursued my formal internship at Loma Linda Medical School University and a full residency program at UCLA (University California at Los Angeles). There was a very smart physician, Dr. Guy Abraham MD, who helped diagnose my problem and taught me how to start magnesium therapy.

Magnesium is a mineral found in soil, and due to modernization in the farming system, it is depleted in our vegetables and fruits. Unfortunately, due to my college lifestyle habit, taking coffee with a false hope of energy and an artificial "lift" from the caffeine, I drained my magnesium faster than I could replenish it. I experienced symptoms of Hypomagnesia syndrome. I have been off coffee since. I healed faster than I thought by supplementing with magnesium at that stage. My skin improved drastically and my hair color returned to my dark brown normal hair. All muscles became stable with less cramping as long as I kept my red blood cell magnesium at a proper level, and I no longer fell asleep in dark places during lectures or movies.

After reading my story probably you may think coffee is bad. Well it has a good taste and the green coffee bean extract contains chlorogenic acid (CGA) which is very bioavailable in humans. It has cinamic acid derivatives that work as antioxidants and anti-inflammatory agents. Caffeoylguinic acid (CqA) and dicaffeoylguinic acid (diCQA) were studied, and the data in humans were nonexistent. The *Journal of Evidence Based Complementary and Alternative Medicine* 2013 18:309–213 shows that 30 percent of these acids were found in urine excretions; therefore it is bioavailable.

The news about green coffee bean extract was so high, that I could not believe that a prominent MD (medical doctor) speaker from UCLA discussed it in front of more than 10,000 medical doctors who love to drink coffee and the response during a pre-med conference in 2014 was very warm. The speaker gave a disclaimer that they were not working for Starbucks nor receiving commissions from coffee bean and tea leaf distributors. The conclusion was it also helps to regulate high blood pressure, but more studies are needed to prove this point. I am glad that something good comes from this delicious but dangerous drink for us.

This may explain why the number one disease in the orthopedic field is osteoporosis. Why would people, who go to their doctor every year and be told to take calcium for their bones and also eat bananas for their potassium content, still suffer osteoporosis and also gain unexpected weight after menopause? Coffee tends to extract the magnesium from our bodies and removes it through the urine. The acidity in coffee is detrimental to our health.

This Western lifestyle has spread all over the world. Attending business meetings, waking up in the morning, studying for exams, and driving long distances: all of these activities seem to have *coffee* as their constant companion. I still remember that we had to wait to drink coffee until our 21st birthday, just like alcohol. But now children are given sweet coffee drinks that are available everywhere and by their own parents. You can simply pick up pre-mixed coffee drinks with tons of sugar in an eight-ounce bottle as a drink for consumption.

Talking about coffee, caffeine or magnesium, doctors like Dr. Guy Abraham have dedicated their time to this subject and written double-blind studies and published in peer-reviewed, prestigious journals more than a dozen times. After a few years of hard work, Dr. Abraham's magnesium protocol which initially was called Voo

Doo or non-EBM (Evidence-Based Medicine) appears neatly in the conventional OBGYN book for medical students. Its indication includes treating eclampsia and pre-eclampsia patients. This is to save both the mothers and the babies during pregnancy and deliveries. His conclusion was pregnant mothers who drink coffee need more magnesium and perhaps should avoid all acidic drinks with caffeine.

To me, this is very fascinating because I went to a conventional medical school yet I bumped into something like this before its birth in conventional practice. I had high interest in exploring natural medicine as well as acupuncture and herbology. These protocols have been used for thousands of years by Asians and particularly the Chinese in China. I pursued this field and researched into the filed from experienced doctors in this field. My first journey into my Integrative Medicine education was very fortunate because of Dr. Abraham's advice. I joined ACAM (American College of Advancement in Medicine) and learned so much about detoxification (homotoxicology) and intravenous nutrients and chelation protocols. I enjoyed every minute, and I felt like I was in a Disneyland of real medical "miracles."

Yet I found out also that the world was still focusing on conventional therapy as they are fixated on double-blind studies. One of the best observations I made was a cardiac bypass operation. This procedure was never given a double-blind study. Whoever the first patient was, was actually the guinea pig of this procedure. Each patient becomes the study field of the cardiac surgeon. Since there can be no double-blind studies on cardiac bypasses, doctors are operating, hoping it will work based on experience. How about Human Growth Hormone (HGH) therapy, which often is called a hoax. It is called that by ignorant doctors or people who are waiting for a double-blind study on HGH. I would not want to be one of the double-blind study patients, thinking I would get some new therapy but being not exactly sure whether I was actually receiving it because it is a blind study.

My interest in Integrative Medicine was unstoppable as I learned more about all kinds of nutrition that heal diseases. People's interest was so persistent that in 1990 the terminology of vitamins changed. It varied from time to time until it becomes a "nutraceutical." It means a nutritional supplement with pharmaceutical effects. They are food-based but have medicinal values just like pharmaceutical drugs. We use this to help patients with a very low risk of getting any side effects unless they are allergic to the food itself. These patients can be tested for delayed reaction allergies that can be treated also with a natural program.

Since then, I focus on studying how to formulate this nutraceutical so I prescribe fewer and fewer drugs when I can use nutraceuticals instead. The name is nutraceutical (nonprescription) or some call it "medical food" that requires a prescription to purchase it. Most medical food is priced right for the patients.

In this book chapters, I want to mention as well that, without my family support, it would be hard to be different than what is expected by the medical community. This goes to my parents, husband, and children. They are the most involved and have helped me from day one until today. I wish they worked in my office as they already know how I think and work. I want people to do what I do, investing in health and their family's health before anything else. It is now possible with Integrative Medicine as you are not just taking drugs but building a stage of healthy aging.

Summary

I tell you from now on that you can have a comprehensive annual physical exam where you have numbers in your blood test to see how you can:

1. Prevent major medical illnesses like stroke, and cardiac events that usually come as a thief in the night.
2. Tell you that you need a change in your lifestyle.
3. See what kind of food you should avoid if it has caused an inflammatory effect on your immune system
4. Know if the cheapest baby aspirin works well with your platelets. Discover pills that have no risk or negative side effects and are not a toxic chemical mix tablet.

5. Show why you are stressed or feel anxiety that comes and goes or why suddenly there is a migraine or psychiatric disorder where no family history existed.
6. Show you why you are moody and how you can have a peaceful solution without having to worry about side effects. Also we can show you how to prevent osteoporosis, chronic fatigue syndrome, and adrenal fatigue.
7. See if you need to repair your gut before it takes you to the hospital and do an endoscopy and colonoscopy just to see if anything is wrong because you have constipation.
8. See if your bottles of supplements in the cupboard are duplicates so you won't overdose and save money.
9. Prevent diabetes that is still in the pre-diabetes stage.
10. See why you accumulate fat and can't lose weight, no matter what.

This list can expand depending on the symptoms you come in with. In our office, we see people who look nice and healthy but with goals like those listed above. They want to prevent sickness common to Americans and remain healthy all their lives. Due to the ignorance of the medical field today, people are just seeing doctors when they are sick. Sometimes it is too late to recover fully.

Our way of testing and interpretation is preventive as well as therapeutic. Interpreting the numbers and combining them to make sense to both doctors and patients are the keys in the success of holistic medicine. Aging is inevitable, but prevention is vital to healthy aging. Since we are all subjected to the current polluted cities and countries in general, our bodies are compensating more. Instead of waiting until the body organs fail, the holistic doctors will try to find a solution to help them compensate before illness sets in. We know that statistics show the majority of the diseases are from the aging process itself. We now know that we can slow down this process and reverse it in many conditions.

Over thirty years ago when I entered my internship training, they were talking about *telomerase* and how to test this so we know if we were aging too fast. A few years ago, we found a way to test it and also now have products that can reverse the aging of the telomeres in our DNA. Staying young and healthy is a key to being a successful person. This integrative holistic approach is a combination of serious complex matters. Most patients will be surprised to see how much they can learn about their own body.

ANTI-AGING MEDICINE

I really love this name. It sounds very sexy and makes people's eyebrows raise and begin checking their faces to see if they need anything. Since Sheldon Hendler PhD MD, and national/international visionaries Ronald Klaz DO and Robert Goldman DO with their Academy of Anti-Aging Medicine (A4M). It is the latter one that I joined. Since the inception of their company, I worked as a volunteer nonpaid physician in education and board examiner, I learned how to apply this to my practice. They are one of the oldest, besides the American College of Advancement in Medicine (ACAM), who produce competent Integrative Medicine doctors. Many other respectful associations like International Functional Medicine by Jeffery Blend PhD, or American Holistic of Integrative Medicine and many dozens of others who are in active operation, as they grow with people interested in this field.

Those who are not an MD or DO can also join this association to learn alternative management in their own field. Other health professionals involved are nutritionists, nurse practitioners, physician assistants, naturopathic doctors, chiropractic doctors, doctors of physical therapy, and all postgraduate professionals in the medical field.

I love to see all of them there as they seem to relate to the population and consumers best as they usually contribute the most to the practical issues and are not contaminated by their previous schools or by Big Pharma products. All of us seem to be happier doctors and health professionals, knowing that we can help the population without worrying about the negative side effects of our recommendations. It is a blessing that Integrative Medicine was approved last year and will continue to grow in knowledge and technology as both conventional and integrative medicine grow side by side.

Many people think the anti-aging name is misleading. I understand their point. We all grow older. I like the name because it was the initial name that started the whole integrative medical movement and made changes in conventional medicine. The name sounds correct for people who already understand how it works. This name creates an immediate assumption that it has something to do with facial improvement so you can look younger. Often their first question is "Do you do Botox injections?" Currently, with the finding of measuring our telomerase, the anti-aging meaning will be more suitable especially when we can show the way to reverse the length of the telomase and slow aging.

In my office we offer aesthetic medicine where we also apply natural nontoxic and nonchemical ingredients to their face to improve the skin condition or fine wrinkles. It has nothing to do with surgical facelift like the plastic surgeons do. For science-based purposes, many other terms are used, such as *reversing senescence*, meaning reversing biological changes in our body. Using some laboratory testing, we can show the physical changes. Improving these markers means making the person feel better and younger. Your ability to stay healthy in your lifetime is often addressed as longevity. This is used also when you talk to common people where they are used to hearing this, and they immediately associate this with "good long life."

Although I have been practicing Integrative Medicine, I have called it in the past both anti-aging medicine or integrative interchangeably. The latter one seems to confused people. They do not know how to integrate this with the conventional medicine. People better understand the terms *conventional* or *traditional*.

INTEGRATIVE MEDICINE

Integrative Medicine is the practice of combining the conventional knowledge to the selection of evidence, based on alternative medicines available. Those practitioners who are trained to understand an integrative approach and laboratory testing can identify the problems far earlier if any are detected in our system. In this approach, the physician is focusing on the whole system or body. By doing so, they can find the cause of the patient's complaint. This integrative approach does not necessarily use the end medication that is usually prescribed to kill the symptoms, but they may use something that fills the deficit in the natural element in our body.

In other words we address the cause, not just the symptoms. Usually we do not use the pharmaceutical, FDA-approved drugs with their side effects. Instead, we use a pharmaceutical with a natural base while following FDA regulations because they do not produce negative side effects. Most of the issues can be handled by the use of natural medication or alternative medicine rather than the prescription pharmaceutical drugs. However, since we are also are medical doctors or doctors of osteopathic medicine, we can at any time use the conventional drugs to start or in combination as may be needed.

Around 50–100 years ago, people learned how to take vitamins. To differentiate from this, we don't use this terminology because vitamins are one only among many other nutraceutical products.

NUTRACEUTICAL

This terminology started back in 1990 where nutrition was used in certain doses to create pharmaceutical effects. They are not just vitamins but include minerals, amino acids, proteins, herbal blends, or even a cocktail of many vitamins and minerals given in the muscles or intravenously.

Lately, for the past two or three years, Big Pharma, which has been monopolizing the drug industry in the world, has also produced some nutraceutical products, and they have started using terminology like "medical food." They are mixing some of the strong ingredients (chemical mix) that have fewer side effects or none to be approved by the FDA. They are asking physicians to write prescriptions for them. Most of them are very expensive, but insurance companies still would cover only a partial cost of this. The pharmaceutical company involved might print many coupons and limit the amount of copayment so patients can afford this mixture of medical food.

It is very difficult to claim 100 percent natural and toxin-free when some of the minerals contain a small percentage of lead (heavy metal) that if taken in a large amount can be harmful. FDA quickly tightens these regulations to make sure the labeling says this has not been evaluated by them and can be harmful to your health. I am just hoping by doing correct labeling, the patients understand how hard and difficult it is for the Integrative Medicine industry to survive. They finally are populating 50 percent of the medication sales in America for the first time. You can feel this, as current pricing is very competitive. Places like a discounted pharmacy also want a piece of the action and are selling these in big volume like Costco, big-volume, discounted stores in America. The pharmacies would carry them over the counter. This competition results in many good ways for our patients to get these products since not every one of them can afford to see an integrative medicine expert, especially when they do not have any health insurance to cover themselves. Books like this would be their guide to understanding how to self-treat and not spend unnecessary money to overlap what they do not need.

This Book will assist you to see usage of nutraceuticals in three categories of the aging process. Stages are divided by four categories, based on clinical symptoms and patient's complaints

PRECLINICAL STAGE (20–40 years of age)

First is for those who just have entered what we call, the *preclinical stage*. Most of them are in the beginning of a declining stage of hormonal production and entering their busy life and are under stress to thrive better in the family. They are usually between the ages of twenty and forty years. They usually have no apparent clinical symptoms yet but have symptoms like tiredness, less stamina, and less ability to exercise; they are less flexible or are unable to work long hours. They are not worried about wrinkles or losing hair yet. They are in what we would call a premature aging stage of these categories.

CLINICAL STAGE (40–60 years of age)

The next categories might need different testing or laboratories checks since this is called the *clinical phase* (ages 40–60). Most patients start to show some clinical signs. As I wrote in my previous book, you might see this one as the transition phase, but in reality and based on my clinical observation, they are really in a clinical stage.

Many people are concerned as their mom or older family members aged much later than they, with those wrinkles, sagging skin, marked hormonal changes, menopause with short pre-menopausal period, lower sexual functions, grey hair, thinning hair, and organ system disturbances like gassy stomach, bloating and some constipation. Also now, ailments like insomnia, getting stressed easily, and sometimes being drug dependent or diagnosed with a real disease such as diabetes, chronic urinary infection, prostate enlargement, and increased frequency of urination are typical. Many have started having cancer, stroke, and cardiovascular insults in this stage.

This population apparently is the most subject to stress in the financial area, especially if they are already married and have children. Most of them, who come to my clinic, have some sort of stress factors, such as a divorce situation, separation from family, or death of their parents.

ADVANCED STAGE OF AGING (60–80 years of age)

These patients are between sixty and eighty years old. They might not have the same stressors as the previous stage. In this population, they are usually wiser and arrive in my office with a reasonably healthy situation by their own definition. If they have symptoms, this population has inherited some prescription medication by their primary physician who managed to see them annually at least to maintain their health by conventional measures. Most come because they have symptoms that can no longer be solved by taking their medications, and they seek solutions with many fewer side effects. They also would love to maintain their previous stage of activities, which they have lost with their aging conditions.

This population may have severe baldness, typical wrinkles that they don't mind anymore, eye problems—either cataracts or floaters or glaucoma—that they think are inevitable and cannot be prevented. They may wake up at night while developing less and less energy and insomnia. They are retired from their main job but usually are still actively doing some hobbies or are working to survive by moonlighting for income to supplement their social security income.

Many come with hypertension, diabetes, chronic fatigue, chronic fibromyalgia syndrome, weakness, loss of partial or full sexual functions and, worse, some come with a stressful diagnosis of cancer. Many come when cancer has advanced to stage 3 or 4, and they could not tolerate the side effects of chemo. Heavy metal toxic syndrome is common, and hypothyroidism is found in almost 80 percent of this population.

LONGEVITY STAGE/PRE-CENTENARIAN (80–100)

They are the winners, as they have maintained a reasonably healthy active life at more than eighty years old, and I see them from eighty to one hundred years old in my office. They are the best to work with as they know how important it is to remain active. However, their financial situation does not allow them to luxuriously enjoy an integrative approach since they have adjusted their lifestyle considerably. They will thrive when they come without major diseases. Those who came to me in the previous stage and carried on to this stage are very happy and feel blessed by routinely doing my prescribed program

Integrative Medicine should always integrate both conventional and alternative, back and forth. At a certain age when organs fail due to certain genetic factors, we need to put them in the hospital for urgent or emergency management. They can get all kinds of appropriate help there, but hopefully when they come out, my integrative medicine approach will restore their health. Most of this population is happy if their family is accompanying them to our place. It reduces their stress by having family members drive them to our office at the age of 100 or so.

I hope all centenarians, the last group, can still be very active, but due to the apparent aging symptoms, they need special protection.

CENTENARIAN STAGE (100+ years)

This is last stage at the top of the pyramid of the population.

In China, there is a city called Su Chou, and during my visit last year, I witnessed how the advanced-stage centenarian population is walking around, doing their errands. They are bicycling, and you wouldn't guess that they are more than 100 years old. They attribute their longevity to the water they have from their mountain. I need to do more research on these centenarians and discover all the secrets—besides their genes.

Here you can see the latest life expectancies table.

WHO—World Health Organization Healthy life Expectancy (DALE), United Nations Statistic Division, trends and statistics 200. Life expectancy and Infant mortality; National Center for Health Statistic—NCHS 1998.

Life expectancy is defined as the average maximum age a person expects to reach. This is derived by some calculation of the average maximum lifespan of persons alive in the whole population.

I am writing in this book all my understanding, based on my thirty years of practicing Integrative Medicine and their results plus my own research. Other books might come later with specific topics like the diseases named or each of the age stage categories. However for practical purposes, this book is about knowledge that people of all ages can benefit from. However, unless they follow all the steps, the chance of slowing down their aging is not optimal.

Those steps are:

1. Detoxification in many systems and all phases

2. Proper diet and nutritional supplementation
3. Identifying stress and contra-stress management
4. Supervised balancing of hormone or replacement therapy
5. Safe exercises, according to your stage.
6. Early stage of disease detection and proper treatment
7. Annual comprehensive checkup to maintain healthy aging

Those are the steps that are going to dominate this book.

Chapter 2

THE GENESIS OF HEALTHY AGING

FROM VERIFIED ARTICLES IN WIKIPEDIA, YOU CAN enjoy the number of those centenarians who lived beyond 130 years of age. There is a list of countries that reported and verified those ages of their longevity citizens. The oldest person whose age was verified by modern standards was Jeanne Calment, who lived to 122. The cases in this list include both semi-legendary personages and people whose existence is not doubted.

Hebrew Bible

In the Hebrew Bible, the Torah, Joshua, Job, and 2 Chronicles mention individuals with lifespans up to the 969 years of Methuselah. If we think they were mistaking lunar cycles for solar ones, this would turn an age of 969 "years" into a more reasonable 969 lunar months, or 78½ years of the Metonic cycle.

Some biblical scholars state that, in one view, man was originally to have everlasting life, but as sin was introduced into the world by Adam, its influence became greater with each generation and God progressively shortened man's life. The biblical upper limit of longevity was categorized by the Bible scholar Watchman Lee. He writes we have undergone four successive plateaus of 1,000, 500, 250, and finally 120 years. Others said that before Noah's flood, a "firmament"over the earth (Genesis 1:6–8) contributed to people's advanced age.

Interestingly, the Bible had only one mention of a woman regarding her age. Abraham's wife Sarah is the only woman in the Old Testament whose age is given. She was 127 (Genesis 23:1).

Hinduism

Bhishma among the Hindus is believed to be immortal. His life spanned four generations and considering that he fought for his great-nephews in the Mahabharata War who were themselves in their seventies and eighties, it is estimated that Bhishma must have been between 130 and 370 years old at the time of his death.

Devraha Baba (d. 1990) was rumored to be over 700 or even over 750 years old.

Islam

According to 19th-century scholars, Abdul Azziz al-Hafeed al-Habashi lived 673/674 Gregorian years or 694/695 Islamic years, from 581–1276 of the Hijra.

Below is a list of living super centenarians. There are forty-eight such individuals, of whom forty-six are female and two are male.

Rank	Name	Sex	Birth date	Age as of 22 August 2015	Place of residence
1	Susannah Mushatt Jones[1]	F	6 July 1899	116 years, 47 days	United States
2	Emma Morano[1]	F	29 November 1899	115 years, 266 days	Italy
3	Violet Brown[1]	F	10 March 1900	115 years, 165 days	Jamaica[a]
4	Anonymous[1]	F	15 March 1900	115 years, 160 days	Japan
5	Nabi Tajima[1]	F	4 August 1900	115 years, 18 days	Japan
6	Kiyoko Ishiguro[1]	F	4 March 1901	114 years, 171 days	Japan
7	Chiyo Miyako[1]	F	2 May 1901	114 years, 112 days	Japan
8	Dominga Velasco[1]	F	12 May 1901	114 years, 102 days	United States[b]

The Genesis of Healthy Aging

Rank	Name	Sex	Birth date	Age as of 22 August 2015	Place of residence
9	Towhee Yorimitsu	F	30 September 1901	113 years, 326 days	Japan
10	Eudoxie Baboul	F	1 October 1901	113 years, 325 days	France (French Guiana)
11	Matsudo Kageyama	F	10 October 1901	113 years, 316 days	Japan
12	Emma Otis[1]	F	22 October 1901	113 years, 304 days	United States
13	Ana Maria Vela Rubio	F	29 October 1901	113 years, 297 days	Spain
14	Mistune Toyoda	F	15 February 1902	113 years, 188 days	Japan
15	Marie-Josephine Baudette	F	25 March 1902	113 years, 150 days	Italy[c]
16	Yukie Hino[1]	F	17 April 1902	113 years, 127 days	Japan
17	Giuseppina Projetto	F	30 May 1902	113 years, 84 days	Italy
18	Goldie Michelson[1]	F	8 August 1902	113 years, 14 days	United States[d]
19	Anonymous[1]	F	7 September 1902	112 years, 349 days	Japan
20	Kiyo Oshiro	F	15 September 1902	112 years, 341 days	Japan
21	Helen Wheat[1]	F	16 September 1902	112 years, 340 days	United States
22	Massa Isère	F	19 September 1902	112 years, 337 days	Japan
23	Masayo Ito[1]	F	1 October 1902	112 years, 325 days	Japan
24	Ethel Farrell[1]	F	27 November 1902	112 years, 268 days	Australia[e]
25	Adele Dunlap[1]	F	12 December 1902	112 years, 253 days	United States

Rank	Name	Sex	Birth date	Age as of 22 August 2015	Place of residence
26	Kane Tanaka[1]	F	2 January 1903	112 years, 232 days	Japan
27	Gladys Hooper[1]	F	18 January 1903	112 years, 216 days	United Kingdom
28	Irene Ciuffoletti	F	19 January 1903	112 years, 215 days	United States[f]
29	Elizabeth Delaney[1]	F	12 March 1903	112 years, 163 days	United States
30	Yasutaro Koide	M	13 March 1903	112 years, 162 days	Japan
31	Tsuto Hori	F	15 March 1903	112 years, 160 days	Japan
32	Maria-Giuseppa Robucci	F	20 March 1903	112 years, 155 days	Italy
33	Yasuno Kawamoto	F	15 April 1903	112 years, 129 days	Japan
34	Iso Nakamura	F	23 April 1903	112 years, 121 days	Japan
35	Élisabeth Collot[1]	F	21 June 1903	112 years, 62 days	France
36	Sina Hayes[1]	F	27 June 1903	112 years, 56 days	United States
37	Alida Victória Grubba Rudge[1]	F	10 July 1903	112 years, 43 days	Brazil
38	Tae Ito[1]	F	11 July 1903	112 years, 42 days	Japan
39	Honorine Rondello[1]	F	28 July 1903	112 years, 25 days	France
40	Ila Jones[1]	F	21 August 1903	112 years, 1 day	United States
41	Emilia Zucchetti[1]	F	28 August 1903	111 years, 359 days	Italy
42	Hatsuno Goto[1]	F	1 September 1903	111 years, 355 days	Japan
43	Aino Matsuoka[1]	F	3 September 1903	111 years, 353 days	Japan

The Genesis of Healthy Aging

Rank	Name	Sex	Birth date	Age as of 22 August 2015	Place of residence
44	Mélanie Leblais[1]	F	4 September 1903	111 years, 352 days	France
45	Tane Shimada[1]	F	25 September 1903	111 years, 331 days	Japan
46	Shino Mori[1]	F	9 November 1903	111 years, 286 days	Japan
47	Ivy Frampton[1]	F	22 November 1903	111 years, 273 days	United Kingdom
48	Shingo Kitamura[1]	M	18 March 1904	111 years, 157 days	Japan

According to one source, the *Daily News*, they have written this about the approximate number of centurion and super centenarians in the future:

> The number of people over 100 years old will reach 110,000 by 2037: Growing life expectancy means number of over-80s will reach six million by the same year.

> Based on their investigations these super centenarians are not on prescription drugs, and their daily lifestyle is very nonabusive, and they maintain moderate amounts of a healthy diet that gives them good nutrition.

> Genetic factors plays 30 percent; however 70 percent are environmental influences. These two interact together and influence each other in specific ways.

Looking at those numbers of a premodern metropolitan world, we can draw many conclusions of why Integrative Medicine will play the most important role in keeping people healthy and functional.

I also would like to touch on the study done by one of the famous gerontologists in United States, the late Dr. Nathan Shock, PhD. He is known as one of the fathers of gerontology and has a huge impact on gerontologist practitioners. He has a famous study called the "Baltimore Longitudinal Study of Aging." He concluded, "Aging is not a disease," contrary to the opinions of many other gerontologists.

Current studies of aging are also being conducted by other specialists such as microbiologists, endocrinologists, neurobiologists, medical doctors, doctors of osteopathy, biologists, statisticians, physicists, osteopathic and oriental medical doctors, acupuncturists, herbologists, and even environmentalists.

We are living in a period of modern medicine, and in order for us to understand fully, we have to be very open-minded, as aging and longevity go hand-in-hand with biological chemicals, psychological influence, and social economy of the patients. Likewise the countries, spiritual situations of the person, the society, and political behaviors or turmoil all create a shift in medicine and its handling or management of the aging population.

If the primary care physician, the specialist, or any of us ignore the above essential elements that support longevity, I don't think the numbers of centenarians will be improved. For example, all the wars in the past have created disasters and toxic environments that affected the health of the populations and their children. The worst examples are where a nuclear weapon was launched, such as that dropped on Hiroshima or where biological weapons were used, such as those used on the Kurds in Iraq.

When I was in my internship, I saw that post-traumatic disorder syndrome and Agent Orange syndrome were being questioned. Not too many people understood those afflictions. That was thirty years ago. Nowadays, I still am examining those veterans of the wars, and you can see clearly which war produces which kind of diagnosis or illnesses. It took three decades for the system to acknowledge the existence of these conditions that affect aging tremendously in one's life.

Those Chinese, Tibetans, Indian Baddish, and Hindus might not have been involved in the study of longevity, but they have used longevity techniques and exercises to slow down their premature aging and also to expedite any healing processes. The Chinese use herbal sand that was considered a tea in the past. Amazon doctors (those wiccans and witches) have mastered the amazon mix or herbal mix which affects longevity. I have learned this from my own patients who told me about what they eat and what they do at home. Many of them are isolating themselves from food that is sold in the market, and they grow their own vegetables and fruits and also mix their own medicines from natural leaves and roots found in their own garden. I am impressed.

One of the keys to understand why all of this comes so slowly is because aging is a slow process that is not supposed to be like all diseases. It is a blessing that it grows slowly because our economy would collapse if the changes were fast. We have to think how we are going to afford all the older people who will need more help in the near future. Strong family culture will definitely help. It has been reflected since the genesis of man, where the children would be raised and trained by their parents or elderly, and later on, they would be taken care by their children as they age. This assurance from the family has a great impact on one's longevity. Western allopathic or conventional medicine embrace gerontologist's study as the process of aging as a disease. This is the big difference from the Integrative Medicine physician who would treat aging not as a disease but a natural process. In 1984 the MacArthur Foundation study has pointed this out.

Allopathic Western conventional medicine sees the pathology and symptoms of aging. They focus on objective studies or laboratories, and this leads them to naming aging as a diagnosis of a sickness, not natural aging. But Integrative Medicine works on prevention and improvement of physiological function to get rid of the cause of diseases, not by just treating the symptoms. It would be best if every field in our Western medicine inserted this education into all conventional medicine training. It would even be best if at one point, every doctor who is practicing would have a background in Integrative Medicine.

My friends and one niece are doctors of osteopathy which are reciprocated as medical doctors in the United States. But in reality, the DO (doctor of osteopathy) studies extra subjects called clinical kinesiology. Although the knowledge was introduced in preclinical studies of medical schools, due to financial considerations, the medical schools did not continue emphasizing this as important. In other words, drugs pay more and are easier to patent.

The DO would be the expert of craniosacral adjustment, and she helps patients with certain symptoms such as migraine or chronic headache or spine malfunction which suits Integrative Medicine.

The Okinawan centenarian studies would be the most interesting studies for the Western people. You can read about this in the book *The Okinawan Program* by Bradley Wilcox, MD (2001). And the university where I studied, UCLA, have mammalian models that are used to study the aging process. This is also done in Berkeley and in other state universities like the University Arizona in Tucson. Monkeys (macaque, rhesus, and squirrel monkeys) are available to be used as they are the closest mammals to humans.

Chapter 3

The History of Medicine

Time line of medicine

2600 BC   The Egyptians established diagnosis and treatments.

460 BC   Birth of Hippocrates, the Greek father of medicine, began to study the performance of a medication similar to aspirin.

300 BC   Diocles wrote the first anatomy book.

130 AD   Galen, Greek physician to gladiators and Roman kings

60 AD   First metria medican written by Pedanius Diocorides.

910   Thazes identifies small pox—Persian.

1489   Leonardo Da Vinci dissects corpses.

1590   Zacharius Jannssen invents the microscope.

1683   Anton Van Leeuwenhoek observes bacteria.

1763   Caludius Aymand performs the first successful appendectomy

1857	Louis Pasteur identifies germs as cause of disease
1849	Elizabeth Blackwell is the first woman to gain a medical degree in Geneva Medical College in New York.
1870	Robert Koch and Louis Pasteur establish the germ theory of diseases.
1895	Wilhelm Conrad Roentgen discovers X-rays.
1899	Felix Hoffman develops aspirin.
1901	Karl Landsteiner introduces Blood type system A, AB, O, and B.
1921	Edward Melanby discovers that lack of Vitamin D in the diet causes Ricketts disease.
1922	Insulin first use to treat diabetes
1928	Sir Alexander Fleming discovers penicillin.
1945	First vaccine for influenza
1950	John Hopkins invented first cardiac pacemaker.
1952	Jonas Salk develops first vaccine for polio.
1963	Thomas Fogarty invented balloon embolectomy catheterization.
1964	First vaccine for measles
1967	First vaccine for mumps
1970	First vaccine for rubella

The History of Medicine

1974   First vaccine for chicken pox

1975   Robert Sledley invents CAT scans

1977   First vaccine for pneumonia

1978   First test-tube baby was born

1981   First vaccine for hepatitis B

1983   HIV virus first identified

1984   Alec Jeffrey found genetic fingerprinting method

1985   Willem J Koff invented artificial kidney dialysis.

1992   First vaccine for hepatitis A

1996   Dolly the sheep as a first clone

2006   The first vaccine targeting the cause of cancer

As you can see, the information presented here is not as complete as it should be, but at least we know what kind of findings influenced the world as medicine changes.

There were other divisions, such as prehistoric medicine from which there was no recorded story about how the herbal leaves become medicines, making it hard to trace. But after the antiquity era, there is more specific information due to the written findings. Those were from Egypt, the Middle East, India, China, and Greek medicine. No one asked about double-blind studies then, and everyone was still improving. They all sought the same goal: healthy aging.

After that comes Hippocrates, the Greek Father of Medicine, which covered the Celsius, Alexandria, and Galen eras.

Islamic and Middle Eastern medicines were established in the 9th and the 12th centuries.

Medieval Europe, in 400–1400 AD, was when we started formal schools and there were theaters and comedians.

The Renaissance era was the early modern period and covered the 16–18th centuries. We had Paracelsus, Padua, and Bologna, women in medicine, Age Enlightenment, and the Britain involvement.

In the 19th century began the rise of modern medicine. There were significant findings, such as the germ theory and bacteriology. Women became more involved as both nurses and physicians.

Paris, Vienna and Berlin led in modern medicine.

The statistical method began to be applied during the US Civil War.

In the 20th centuries, we see World War I, when public health was introduced, and then in the Second World War, Nazi and Japanese medicine were in high demand.

After that, we had the Post-World War II era where modern surgery was introduced. Medicine continues to improve, and hopefully we can learn from our mistakes. It is about time for us to put all good things together and use them all to improve our public health.

Chapter 4

The Wisdom of Healthy Aging

Just last week, I went to listen to a sermon from my pastor, Fr. Paul Fitzgerald, who I respect in his knowledge, at my parish church, and he was talking about the difference between knowledge and wisdom. It was fascinating. I never thought of differentiating these two. I think that we have to develop that idea. However, I believe that wisdom is a gift that you may or may not receive, depending on your own decisions.

Wisdom is there and given to everyone, but the person has to be open to receive it and to learn how to receive it. Wisdom requires the use of knowledge, but you need to digest the knowledge and develop your own understanding. Isn't that interesting?

The "Word of Wisdom" is the common name of a section of the *Doctrine and Covenants*, a book considered by many churches within the Latter Day Saint movement to consist of revelations from God. It is also the name of a health code, based on their teachings, practiced most strictly by The Church of Jesus Christ of Latter day Saints (LDS Church) and Mormon fundamentalists, and to a lesser extent, some other Latter Day Saint denominations. They have certain health prohibitions like not drinking coffee, tea, or alcohol. Why is it interesting in this context of the book? I have observed for almost thirty years now that I have given a health program to patients who seem to understand the whole concept because they grasp the wisdom of the program and not just the facts or knowledge. It works for these people.

The point is that what we teach as integrative doctors will only work if given to people who use wisdom and apply it over a long period of time. Seventh-Day Adventists, for example, are vegetarians and practice healthy eating. As a result, they live longer and are healthier than the normal US population. They accept it and put it in their heart as a part of their culture at this point. They become healthy and reach longevity. So if you have the wisdom to put our teachings into practice, even if you do not have all the full knowledge about it, then you will be successful.

I hope you understand this because it is very important for the practitioners and also the patients themselves. I begin to wonder about those who are so smart but not healthy. Since genetic factors account for only 30 percent of our health and perhaps less, then why are we not seeing more healthy people using this better way of living? Well, there are many factors that affect our health. I will let the spiritual people, such as pastors and priests, work on the spiritual side of health. However, all disease may have a spiritual beginning like bad attitudes, unforgiveness, and festering anger, for example.

For my job, I accept the oath "Do no harm." When you become a doctor and take the oath, only wisdom will help us understand who those are who have aged successfully. Why do you think the centenarians and super centenarians are so happy and live so long? Isn't it obvious if you can live and be active all your life until you close your eyes, it is almost heaven on earth? There are many theories of aging that have been exposed to everyone who desires to follow health issues.

They are:

1. DNA Damage and Repair Theory: DNA works until the strands of DNA cannot repair themselves anymore.
2. Thermodynamic Theory: you can metabolize until it does not work any more.
3. Neuroendocrine Theory is where you have hormonal imbalances or your body stops producing hormones.
4. In the Free Radical Theory, burned-out cells result from oxygen utilization.
5. In Telomere Theory, chromosomes stop duplicating themselves.

6. In Immune Theory, the immune system imbalances or your immune system weakens.

All of these are able to be tested and digested in finding the causes and protocols in treatments. I have been using laboratories and the patient's specimens with good results as the guide to the protocol or treatment plans. Many times, doctors might say everything is okay, Mr. or Mrs. Smith, and I will see you at the next annual physical, but your symptoms are not all right.

If you come to see me in my office, we will run all kinds of tests, according to what you need. When we find out the results and causes, all of this can be overwhelming, and often, the patient can't believe it is their results that I am giving them in our consultation. When we detect the cause, that is when you need to start thinking straight with your own ability and capacity. This is when the "wisdom of health" needs to kick in. Our relationship has to grow in trust of the program and treatment. I will repeat the tests as often as three times per year, or every four months. If you have the courage and trust the program you will improve. With this Wisdom factor in health, I decided that formal traditional advertisement had less value compare to just patients' word of mouth.

I am waiting for other doctors to send patients when they see centenarians aging well in our program. I thank all my patients that have made our practice grow and remain operational for thirty years now. They are my living testimonies, and I am here to help them maintain their health. After a while, I think they become wiser in health knowledge, and they become spokespersons in their communities and family circles. Some of them are doctors themselves who had advised me not to pursue something "holistic" and something with "no evidence-based science." They still seek double-blind studies. Luckily, I have enough wisdom and knowledge of health so I follow my own judgment.

Those professionals in medicine who seem smart yet do not have this wisdom of health are usually not healthy themselves. I am afraid they are going to come back to me and realize that they should have attained wisdom a long time ago. Many of the protocols in Integrative Medicine have some lifestyle changes that sound like your mother's advice. My mother used to tell all of us to rest in the afternoon for two hours and sleep before showering and then wake up ready to eat dinner after that. Then she would make us sit at this big huge long study table for two to three hours. There were seven of us. After that, we were allowed to play for only thirty to sixty minutes. By then it was about 9:00 p.m. By 10:00 p.m., she would say "If you don't go to sleep early and get enough rest you can't grow tall." Does anyone remember anything like that?

I am not sure, how many listened and followed my mom's advice, but I am the tallest among five girls. Of course, my two brothers are also tall because the males are usually taller in Asian families. Now we know that Human Growth Hormone is released between 11:00 p.m. and 3:00 a.m. from the anterior pituitary gland daily. Many of our parents learned from observation, and they liked to pass it on to their children. They used their wisdom. They did not go to medical school, so definitely they learned these good habits from family and friends.

The Bible discourages "strong drink," getting drunk. In some cases, this includes sacramental wine which has been replaced with sacramental water or grape juice. We don't recommend non-medicinal use of tobacco and hot drinks, and meat should be eaten sparingly.

The Mormon scripture also recommends the consumption of herbs, fruits, and grains, as well as grain-based mild drinks. As practiced by the LDS Church, there is no firm restriction relating to meat consumption, but all narcotics and alcoholic beverages are forbidden, including beer. The Mormon Church interprets hot drinks to mean coffee and tea. Coffee and caffeinated tea are going to bind your minerals—especially magnesium. I am living proof as a victim of coffee.

I lecture at a small group of women's retreats, senior citizen homes and halls, and Lions clubs. Included in my presentation, I quote the Christian Bible regarding what I call "anti-aging quotations."

Chapter 5

PROPHETIC HEALTH

PROPHETIC HEALTH WAS A TERM USED DURING THE 13–14th centuries when Islamic religion spread. This therapy consisted of diet and simple drugs (especially honey), bloodletting, and cautery, but no surgery. Other topics included how to handle fevers, leprosy, plague, poisonous bites, protection from night-flying insects, protection against the evil eye, rules for coitus, theories of embryology, proper conduct of physicians, and treatment of minor illnesses such as headaches, nosebleed, cough, and colic. It was prohibited to drink wine or use soporific drugs (commonly known as a sleeping medication or hypnotic medication such as Valium, Ambien) as medications.

Let's see if this is what we want to practice and, not linking health to any specific religions, we know that certain parts of the cities or countries are practicing this religiously. In California, the Adventist Christian follows the "prophetic diet," and many of them are vegetarian. They do not eat pork or shellfish or fish without scales. They don't drink alcohol, coffee, or caffeinated tea, and they are not allowed to smoke cigarettes. Taking Loma Linda as an example of practicing a prophetic diet, their populations have won a mark of longevity in their population of the highest rank. But again, the goal is not to live longer but to live a healthy, long life. Further research and statistics will show if those people also live healthy after all.

I would not want to live a day longer if I have to suffer and stay at home wondering where I am with Alzheimer's or if I have to wait for other people to push me around and feed me. To live longer with severe stroke or brain damage and many other neurological disorders is not our goal. Who wants to live to be 100 years old, and the last of their twenty years are spent suffering from severe gastroenterology problems, such as colitis or irritable bowel syndrome? What about living with chronic fibromyalgia or chronic fatigue disorder? These people cannot enjoy the life they want to live.

Some Buddhists and Taoists practice the same diet and are even more vegetarian than any other religion. They are in an area in northern China which is populated with many centenarians and active, long-living people.

We are in a Western country, and the United States is a land of mixture of religions. However we are a Christian based country because people who first came and discovered America were the Europeans, mostly Christians. In my clinic, I have observed that these populations present the opposite of health. Many of them have a leaky gut, though their prophetic diet does not include meat or pork.

After many years of close observation, the real prophetic diet sounds excellent, but due to the advance in technology and vegetables that are sprayed with pesticide, processed honey, GMO corn, contaminated and medicated stock animals, this prophetic diet has become difficult to follow and trust. To a certain degree, some areas are still clean from toxins but are very rarely found in the United States where most areas are modernized. Basically the best advice for the diet is to eat more organic vegetables and avoid the high glycemic sugar content vegetables that are mostly those grown underground, such as potatoes and carrots, which trigger diabetes and arthritic conditions due to their high glycemic content. Avoid refined sugar and high glycemic grain such as rice or even brown rice. Rice raises our blood sugar levels rapidly like sugar does.

Since Monsanto uses genetically modified crops, such as corn, it is very difficult to find non-GMO corn. Even if they have it, most likely it is sold for higher use in medicine such as injectable vitamin C to help patients who need it the most.

We must avoid artificial sugar that includes aspartame, Splenda, sucralose, and high-fructose corn syrup, which is used everywhere in canned and bottled products on grocery shelves. If you need to use something for a sweet taste, try stevia leaf products which contain no sugar, glucose, agave, or raw honey. Stevia is easily stored in the liver as an energy source instead of going straight into the blood stream, then processed and turned into fat instead of energy.

Encourage your family to stay on a protein content diet of beans and legumes but washed carefully or soaked in water long enough to help our digestive process and cooked well to break down harmful toxins. Some nuts, such as peanuts, contain alpha toxins, and most of them are acidic, except a few like almonds and Brazil nuts. So try to avoid snacking on nuts, as you need to balance your bodily pH from the food you eat.

Organic eggs are good protein, and lean meat from grass-fed animals is an excellent source for protein eaten sparingly. Some people are restricted from eating scavengers. Scavengers are those mentioned in the prophetic diet such as pork, ham, most cured bacon, shellfish, shrimps, lobster, clam, langoustines, and crabs. Again, if you are not restricted by your religion, try to eat less of these as they contain high uric acid levels and may make already-existing arthritis worse.

Soy-based fermented tempeh and miso are both very good sources of protein and are very alkaline. Avoid protein from soy products or soy milk that are processed.

Processing and fermentation destroy the nutrients and original enzymes we need in dairy. Cheese and yogurt in minimal amounts can be tolerated as long as you are not sensitive to dairy.

There is blood testing to find out if you are sensitive to all of these. It is worth it to invest in this esoteric testing as it will save your digestive system which now has become the "port d'entre" (initial passage) for all foods. Autoimmune disease and heart disease can be avoided by proper blood testing for allergies.

There are many other tests to see if your diet agrees with your immune system. Due to high technology, we can test all of these. It makes our job easier and not just a guessing game and making treatment a trial and error program for patients. Diet and nutrition will be discussed in another book or in later chapters. These can be easily confused as the conventional medical doctors never have learned of diet from our medical schools. Dieticians (RDs) also are not taught proper nutrition.

Dieticians learn diets to give to people who are in the hospital or recovering from surgery. Most the time they focus on what they can give them so they transition from liquid to puree and then to their own regular diet. I was surprised to find out what they actually teach at the university level. We are not treating the hospitalized patients properly with good healthy food, so we need to teach regular human beings to eat a proper diet to stay healthy and out of the hospital. Many of our diets are simply "good tasting," but we have to make sure you understand the meaning of moderation in portion size and what the healthy diet is. It is not an easy task to find healthy food in a restaurant, so you must remember when you eat out that the food could be toxic to your body or system.

Many people do not know about allergies that give you a rash on the skin or also cause other symptoms such as dizziness, headache, nausea, joint pain, and muscle stiffness. Most of these "delayed reactions" occur when you can't even remember what you have eaten a few days back. These are the insult called Immunoglobulin G in our systems. These are testable, and it makes it easier to avoid the food that causes inflammatory processes in your body. It is better to be tested and not go through the inflammation process itself.

Although a considerable number of prophetic medicine treatises have been written, we do not have the name of any medical practitioner known for practicing this type of medicine. But it does not matter because we can test the systems and know which foods are not allowed or need to be in moderation. So prophetic or not prophetic are not shown in the result of your blood test. We all know that our body does not involve itself in religion and must be taken care of so you can function in life and be productive instead of staying at home being sick all your life even while eating a prophetic diet.

I am not sure if there is prophetic physician out there who can follow the prophetic diet 100 percent of the time and survive, while taking care of their patient's health. I know about the Jehovah's

Witness physicians who believe that people should not receive blood transfusions during surgery, so they are all trained to keep the patients from losing blood.

I was also informed that the Jehovah's Witness patients who seek elective surgery should seek Jehovah's Witness surgeons. I think that is a need and requires tolerance within reason. If you allow someone to die for lack of blood, that is not a reasonable tolerance to me. But, of course, I am not following the Jehovah Witness laws. I am just a medical doctor who follows the *Do no harm* law.

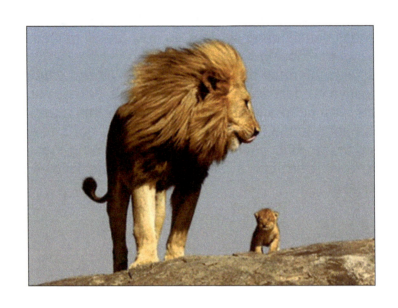

Open My Eyes

God, open my eyes so I may see
And feel your presence close to me.
Give me strength for my stumbling feet
As I battle the crowd of life's busy street,
And widen the vision of my unseeing eyes
So in passing faces I'll recognize
Not just a stranger, unloved and unknown
But a friend with a heart
That is much like my own.
Give me perception to make me aware
That scattered profusely on Life's thoroughfare
Are the best gift of God that we daily pass by
As we look at the world
With an unseeing eyes.
—Helen Steiner Rice

PART TWO

Chapter 6

Introduction — Integrative Medicine: Journey in Healthy Aging

The name *Integrative Medicine* sounds very appropriate but is just the same as Anti-Aging Medicine and other names given to it in the past thirty to forty years. Despite that it has been on my wall of my practice building in Pasadena for years, people are still wondering what it is. I can understand it because people are used to "alternative" more and wonder why that name was not chosen. The reason is because this is not only about alternative medicine.

People who are practicing "alternative medicine" must be well versed in their field such as chiropractic, acupuncture, physical therapy, oxygen therapy; ozone therapy, or naturopathic therapy. Some are using energy therapy, hydrotherapy, urine therapy, fecal transplant, and spiritual therapy. I often witness those who are healed by spiritual therapy and water therapy. Integrative Medicine is a field that combines both conventional medicine and alternative medicine practices.

This field has evolved, and thank God for it. I am so grateful that my previous conventional training gave me the insight that patients can be treated with alternative medicine, but if they have to get some help from a conventional protocol to stabilize their health, it is available, also. We are not talking about one of the other but "Both And." This is exactly how doctors or physicians or practitioners have to meet from both sides of the world.

Doctors in the new system that are approved by the American Board of physicians have to qualify by completing coursework in medical schools or something equivalent. Like Doctors of Osteopathic medicine (DO), Integrative Medicine is an equivalent and carries the same weight or even perhaps more being trained in kinesiology, as we know. These doctors must complete and be board certified in their own recognized specialties credentialed by the ABPS (American Board of Physician Specialty).

According to the newly established regulations, which I am sure will grew in policies as it grows in size, doctors are allowed to attend the two years of formal training in Integrative Medicine. This field has its own Board of Examination for those who are interested in improving their credentials for their practice and boost their own confidence, just like other specialties.

I still remember when I went through specialty medicine after I graduated. Now I understand why I kept changing specialties when I started with OBGYN, which lasted me for only for one month before I embarked in Pediatrics.

Due to my background in an Asian family and in Asia; child abuse reported cases were nonexistent in the hospitals. In some countries, spanking their own children for bad behavior was common, whereas in the United States, you might be charged as a "child abuser" and be put in jail.

You probably are familiar with the above idea as not too long ago we witnessed an American boy who purposely violated Singaporean law of "no littering and graffiti" and was caught spray-painting another person's car. Although he was a minor and an American citizen, the Singaporean government considered that criminal and, with public caning on open skin, punished him. This was a shock to the Americans, and I remember that even our President Bill Clinton pleaded to have him returned and be tried in US law; the plea was turned down.

I believe because of their strict government laws, Singapore is the cleanest city and country in the world. I wonder if we should have stricter laws at work everywhere in the world. I personally have mixed feelings about it.

I was shocked after one night I witnessed seven child abuse cases come to our pediatric emergency department. Not sleeping the whole night is not a problem for me, but given seven severely abused children at the age of five, seven, and nine in one night put me in total culture shock.

I resigned the following week but made the decision when I wrote all those seven case reports that were one-inch thick for each case. Not that I am not capable of handling those cases but I don't think it is fair for my patients to see me as a doctor handling those cases.

I have given you a perfect example above. Doctors need special training to handle certain types of cases. I would also want to tell you that proper training for Integrative Medicine doctors should be established. Too many conventional doctors do not understand and continue telling patients that we refer to them to quit using supplements because they are not prescribed. They even told some of my patients that the supplements we gave them can cause liver and kidney damage if given too much. It is a good thing the majority of my patients are well educated in the Integrative Medicine field by now. In fact, they are much more educated than many conventional doctors about vitamins B or vitamin C or even calcium and minerals.

To my colleagues, who are not well versed in this field, it is good enough that you see the patients and do your best in your field. You can say that you are not well versed in Integrative Medicine, and you tell the patients that you are a medical doctor and well trained in your field. When patients ask questions their doctors can't answer, doctors should refer them to the integrative doctor instead saying this is something they are not trained to do.

I send my patients to a well-mannered cardiologist or gastroenterologist or even OBGYNs and back to their primary physicians for their specific specialty when they are in need of that treatment. I could open my books on my walls and read more about their case and buy extra equipment, I could pretend to know and treat them, but I don't think that is ethical. I know my limits in training, and all doctors should admit that. All of us went through the same training as doctors of medicine, and my thinking is we have to help our colleagues to do "no harm" to their patients. So this principle makes the journey of Integrative Medicine smoother. I attribute the smooth-sailing journey to the patients and population who demand this practice more because we have extra training.

Back to my journey of seeking a good residency program that fits my personality, I ended up taking a psychiatry rotation and then neurology. And it was then that my brother had a stroke, and God showed me another emerging field then called Physical Medicine and Rehabilitation. I completed that training at UCLA, and it was then I found my love to practice, which is Alternative medicine.

This journey started with Advance of Medicine and then Anti-Aging Medicine for the longest time and finally is called "Integrative Medicine." I love this field so much, and I also love to see elderly people become more active or stay active during my care. Taking care of toxic patients with severe gastrointestinal disorders and allergies is just as rewarding as seeing some patients who get rid of their migraines, tinnitus, and being able to eat things that they hadn't for a long time. Some patients, who were so toxic after chemotherapy, recovered faster with detoxification treatments.

Most of my friends who were as confused as me thirty years ago have come back and returned as my patients and good friends. Most patients become friends as during consultation they learn more about me and I learn more about them. It is usually a thirty- to sixty-minute session to just start with a new patients and it might need more hours for a more chronic illness or fatigue syndrome.

The journey of Integrative Medicine is "just beginning to form and be regulated." I am so happy about this because other doctors can now learn that this is not something that they have to be afraid of because it is new.

I have smart friends, who are medical doctors by training, who can't comprehend how this field requires training and full education. One doctor would borrow books and try to learn it himself. He is not healthy, and I think he needs too many things done but he is not willing to find out through the integrative system. Well sure enough, after long years of struggling to occasionally teach him over the phone some protocol and loan him some books, I saw his health deteriorate, I have finally seen his integrative learning improve, and after years, he has come to reverse his aging process. But sometimes it takes a conventional doctor to fail before they can accept that a "preventive measure" is always a better solution for a disease.

An excellent article is about Jim Laidler, "An Alternative-Medicine Believer's Journey Back to Science." by Alan Levinovitz, and an assistant professor of religion at James Madison University.

There are many religion-like aspects to alternative medicine in general. I have seen more in the autistic patients and in treatments called the Bio-med movement. Indeed, it's for good reason that I frequently point out that most "energy medicine" (particularly reiki) is basically faith healing that substitutes Eastern mysticism for Judeo-Christian religious beliefs. I am not qualified to discuss about spiritual miracles or evidence, but I often witness this happening in addition to my conventional treatment for autistic children.

In our office we use the hyperbaric oxygen chamber with mild pressure to lower inflammation and to avoid seizures. This is a miracle in itself when we see the effects in their appetite and other response. Nutrition is most important for autistic children who are very sensitive to milk-casein and gluten-based products. A loving parent is a must, and a skilled speech pathologist is a blessing in this group of needy patients.

Chelation is a big area in Integrative Medicine and has helped autistic children improve should the cause be heavy metal toxicity. Despite that risk, the ADA (American Dental Association) has not banned the use of amalgam in children or even adults as a filler for cavities, but many more wise dentists have decided to not use this material. It is indeed a blessing to see how dentists have become what we call "biological dentists." I am hoping soon that there is a Fellowship for dentists to practice Integrative Dentistry. Although my understanding is just removing some of the "bad batch" protocols and improving knowledge in testing of inflammatory materials and avoiding putting inflammatory metals in our patient's mouths makes them healthier. I have met some specialist dentists who can deal with these problems by using safer protocols.

Gnathology is the study of the masticatory system, including its physiology, functional disturbances, and treatment. It is studied in some dental schools in the United States. However since it is not part of all dental school training, most dentists learn through post-graduate study clubs.

Gnathology is accurate dentistry, verifying the work as it progresses, applying all well-founded gnathological principles, and rechecking the work continually. They are the group that naturally embraces the principles of *do no harm* to our gums and mouth. They use their own degrees that they earned after their training and not the DDS. That really caught my attention. They are the true biological dentists. They do no root canals or other procedures that can cause health issues according to them. They are more knowledgeable about human health in general almost as though they are medical doctors *and* doctors of dental surgery both when they present their points.

I have had the privilege in using Professor Clifford's testing for metals in using a blood sample for almost thirty years now. It started of course with my own problems. I still remember that I was so frightened that I asked my good friend dentist to remove all seven amalgam fillings in my mouth as soon as I found out the horrible things that could happen to my health. Years later, I learned that I was very blessed not to have a detox crisis from removing all seven at once.

My friend was not a biological dentist, but she replaced all seven amalgams and filled the teeth with composite material instead. That was twenty-five years ago. However due to her due diligence, she understood this situation fast, and she has been a biological dentist ever since. Dr. Lillian On DDS has been helping me and my family and patients to have healthy dental care. She has been a biological dentist in our office.

Not long after that, I was very happy to learn that my own sister-in-law recognized that amalgam fillings can be a huge insult when they are placed in our mouth or in our gum line where it can hit high temperatures. When we drink hot coffee and tea, we get the fumes from the amalgams that go into our system and lodge in our fat tissue, brain, bone, and muscles. Students in dental schools, have no choice because amalgam is the cheapest material made available in dental schools. The material arrives with a skull-and-crossbones warning sign, yet they are to use it on their patients. Does that make sense, brothers and sisters?

It has been said that alternative medicine appeals to some unmet need that scientific medicine either does not meet or does a poor job of handling. Whether there is a need for hope when there is little or none or the feeling that "something" is being done, that is perhaps true in many cases. However, unmet psychological needs are not a justification for the acceptance of pseudoscience creeping into conventional medicine. Thus by regulating alternative medicine to Integrative Medicine under the auspices of the medical specialty board, this will ease some of these feelings about the creepy medicine that is used just for financial gain.

If patients choose blindly to hope, and if the providers also blindly use the conventional or alternative medicine approach for patients who hope for a miracle cure without real proven treatment, we all suffer. Sometimes I wonder whether I should write what I learned in conventional medical schools or whether I should write what I think is best based on my knowledge in my clinical experience and practice using a combination approach. The field of Integrative Medicine is considered a baby field, but not a baby science. We are using the ancient and the modern science combination approach for the best of the patient's health.

Needless to say, we have yet to explore scientific-based medicine more and try our best to *do no harm* to our patients. If they have a preference for products or medication that has helped them for a long period, I won't change it unless I know for sure these products or medications have no health benefit for them. It is up to them whether they will follow my advice or continue with something that has not helped them. My job is to tell my patients if there are options but will guide them if there are no options and only hope is left. I have not found an easy way, actually, but I tell them about my previous consistent experience that I use or learn in my continuing medical education courses I take year after year. My goal in this journey is sharing my experiences with newcomers who are interested and also to see healthier next generations to come.

I surely hope that all my friends and relatives will stay healthy and live to an optimal age where we will be in serving the community together. It is a privilege to serve my community and hopefully enjoy healthy aging together.

****

Understanding

Not more of light I ask, O God,
But eyes to see what is;
Not sweeter song, but ears to hear
The present melodies;
Not more of strength, but how to use
The power that I possess:
Not more of love, but skill to turn
A frown to a caress:
Not more of joy, but how to feel
Its kindly presence near
To give to others all I have
Of courage and of cheer.
No other gifts, dear God, I ask,
But only sense to see
How best these precious gifts to use
Thou hast bestowed on me.

—Salesian Mission

Chapter 7

Pillars of Healthy Aging

You wonder what caused your problem but until you understand the Integrative system, I suggest that you try your best to do everything you can to gain optimal health. We all have to agree at one point why we age, and how we age, and what happens when we age. What is I to say that we age too fast or normally and what point do we feel that nothing needs to be done any more as we are at the pyramid of the healthiest condition we can achieve?

Facts about Aging

I use World Health Organization (WHO) reports as they are usually updated.

1. The world population 60–80 "Clinical Stage of Aging"

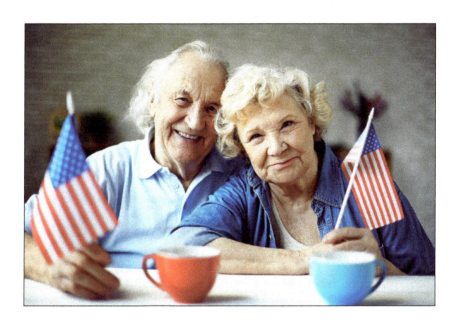

Between 2000 and 2050, the proportion of the world's population over sixty years will double from about 11 percent to 22 percent. The number of people aged sixty years and over is expected to increase from 605 million to 2 billion over the same period.

2. The number of people aged eighty and older (Advanced Stage of Aging) will quadruple in the period 2000 to 2050. By 2050 the world will have almost 400 million people aged eighty years or older. Never before have the majority of middle-aged adults had one living parent.

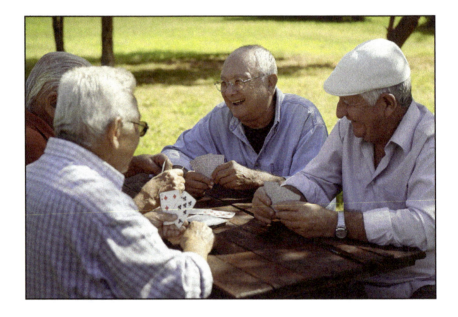

3. By 2050, 80 percent of older people will live in low- and middle-income countries. Chile, China, and the Islamic Republic of Iran will have a greater proportion of older people than the United States of America. The number of older people in Africa will grow from 54 million to 213 million.

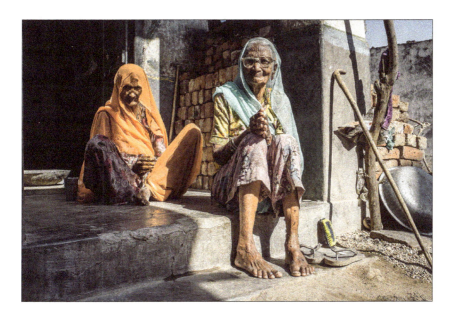

4. The main health burdens for older people are not from communicable diseases.

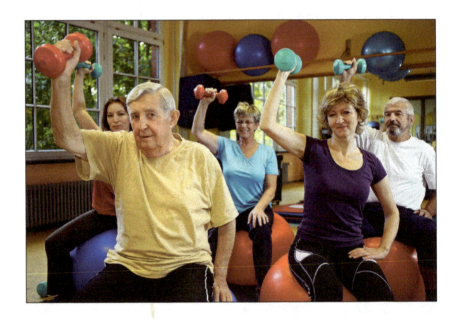

Already, even in the poorest countries the biggest killers are heart disease, stroke, and chronic lung disease, while the greatest types of disability are visual impairment, dementia, hearing loss, and osteoarthritis.

Pillars of Healthy Aging

5. Older people in low- and middle-income countries carry a greater disease burden than those in the rich world.

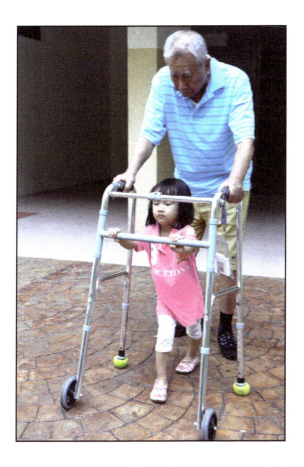

Older people in low- and middle-income countries have around three times the number of years lost to premature death from heart disease, stroke, and chronic lung disease. They also have much higher rates of visual impairment and hearing loss. Many of these problems can be easily and cheaply prevented.

6. The need for long-term care is rising.

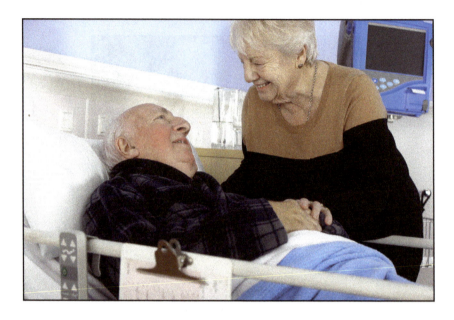

The number of older people who are no longer able to look after themselves in developing countries is forecast to quadruple by 2050. Many of the very old lose their ability to live independently because of limited mobility, frailty, or other physical or mental health problems. Many require long-term care, including home-based nursing, community, and residential and hospital-based care.

7. Effective, community-level primary health care for older people is crucial.

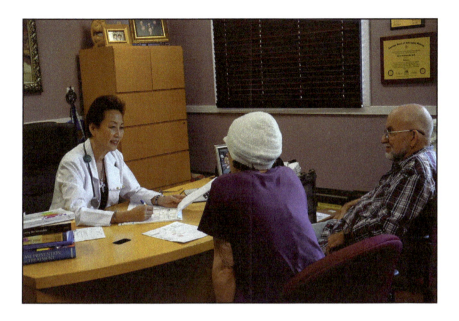

Good care is important for promoting older people's health, preventing disease and managing chronic illnesses. Most training for health professionals does not include instruction about specific care for older people. However, health workers will increasingly spend more of their time caring for this section of the population. WHO maintains that all health providers should be trained on aging issues.

THE NO COAT MEDICINE

8. Supportive, "age-friendly" environments allow older people to live fuller lives and maximize the contribution they make.

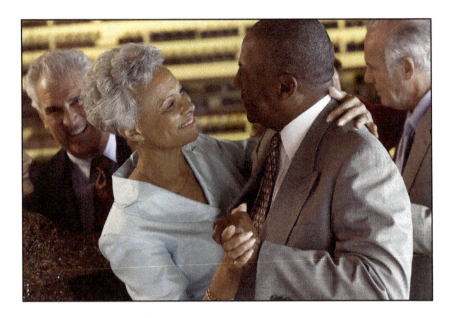

Creating "age-friendly" physical and social environments can have a big impact on improving the active participation and independence of older people.

Pillars of Healthy Aging

9. Healthy aging starts with healthy behaviors in earlier stages of life.

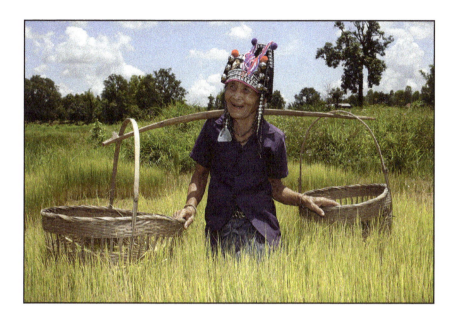

These include what we eat, how physically active we are and our levels of exposure to health risks such as those caused by smoking, harmful consumption of alcohol, or exposure to toxic substances. However, it is never too late to start: for example, the risk of premature death decreases by 50 percent if someone gives up smoking between sixty and seventy-five years of age.

10. We need to reinvent our assumptions of old age.

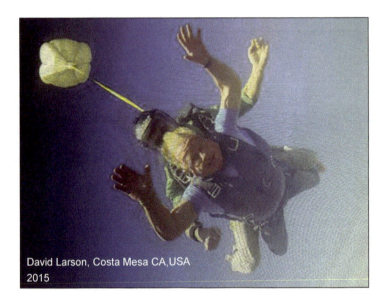
David Larson, Costa Mesa CA, USA
2015

Society needs to break stereotypes and develop new models of aging for the 21st century. Everyone benefits from communities, workplaces, and societies that encourage active and visible participation of older people.

Myths about aging are all over the Internet, and aging is still a scary topic to discuss. Why are people scared? It is due to the aging diseases. Aging itself is not a disease but changes in the physical body and the systems in the body caused by the influences of the environment that create a burden and cause disease that is related to those changes. For conventional doctors to say that "it is only old age and nothing to worry about" when a patient can't sleep at night or has night sweats and has to change their outfit in the middle of the night due to profuse sweating and being soaking wet, is negligence.

Let's go back to the facts. The first death threat of the age related disease is cancer. Five percent of cancers are genetic; 95 percent are preventable in children and adults. Thirty-six percent of cancer cases are diagnosed at the age of seventy-five and over. This statistic is taken from cancer research of the UK and the United States. The rest of cancers are diagnosed between the ages of twenty-five and seventy-five years old.

The increasing occurrence is marked in the last ten years of life, and most of the discussion is linked to environmental issues, diets, and poor hygiene. Not a single source would tell us exactly what causes cancer, but there are indications below and physicians' reports together with the National Health Institute studies. One out of two men and one out of three women will have one type or more cancer in their life.

There are multiples that you can add to the basic pillars, but I like to stay with six of them. It is not too much, and it is not too little so that the important ingredient to healthy aging won't be missed. Obviously to some degree where genetics are involved and chronic diseases have been involved, a special tweak of the pillars must be considered. If the pillar sounds impossible to you, somehow in a mild degree you have to review your own health and visit this pillar at a certain point when your health allows.

For example, if you are very ill, and you can't exercise, then you must wait until there is a slight opportunity. Then you must use the time and carve it out to do some sort of activity called "exercise." Our body needs it, and each of the organs need special attention or certain exercise.

The following are the pillars of healthy aging:

1. Detoxification
2. Diet and nutrition
3. Exercise and Activity
4. Stress Reduction
5. Hormone Balancing
6. Cell regeneration
7. Early Detection of Diseases

Let's begin with the most important pillar, I think, for all ages.

Pillar I
DETOXIFICATION

Your body has a self-built complex detox system. Most of us born healthy have this system in place. It works to detox the environmental toxins or toxins created from our own metabolism and food we eat or air we breathe. Our modern living exposure to more toxins has created an overload burden to normally healthy organs to detox. The burden creates tremendous stress and might cause neuron degeneration and accelerated aging.

The natural detoxification models work when individual cell replacement occurs or tissues are improved with new cells. When this happens, we are at the healthy stage, and this is what is called healthy natural detoxification. The cell tissue cleansing of particles is a therapeutic model for natural detoxification and can be improved with healthy diet and exercise and supplementing with certain antioxidants like vitamin C or B that make our body feel good.

On this topic of the detox pillar I would like to write about the environmental toxins: lead, cadmium, arsenic, aluminum, asbestos and so forth and also the toxins from our diet (pesticides, hormones, antibiotics, and also heavy metals from fish and soils.

Before we discuss the protocol we need to know why it is necessary to detox.

TOXINS CAN SUPPRESS YOUR HEALTH AND IMMUNE SYSTEM

I assume we all know and agree that living in a modern country, we are subject to pollution of the air we breathe, water we drink and use to shower and wash our hair, and the food we eat to nourish our bodies.

The US Environmental Protection Agency's report in the year 2014 showed that progression will grow from an estimated seven billion pounds of toxic waste containing 80,000 different toxic chemicals, including industrial chemicals, drugs, food additives, preservatives, pesticides, herbicides, and xenobiotics have been released in our environment. The list of toxins is available in the Toxics Release Inventory (TRI) Report. It is disturbing enough to hear it and it is worse to see the reports. It seems it gets worse despite what our national team of detoxification tries to do.

That list includes:

1. Air: benzene, gasoline, styrene (styrofoam), toluene (in gasoline)

2. Pesticides: DDT, 1,4 dichlorobenzenes (moth balls and household deodorizers for carpets and air fresheners) and many others

3. Phenols: in our drinking water (ethyl phenol), plastic (bisphenol A. BPA) and others

4. Recreational drugs: cocaine, heroin, amphetamine, and many others

5. Toxic heavy metals: mercury, lead, uranium, cadmium, gadolinium (used in contrast for CT scans or diagnostic radiology), arsenic, aluminum, and thallium

6. Chlorinated organic chemicals: dry cleaning fluids, swimming pool chemicals, and other household cleaners

The excessive amount and accumulation of these substances in our bodies will inhibit the natural process of our body to detoxify and replenish and regenerate again. Most modern pharmaceutical drugs are designed to treat symptoms fast but often cause more toxicity in the body. Many people are aware of this because the regulations have tightened and dispensing drugs has to be accompanied by lengthy information about the side effects of the drugs.

When the detoxification processes are introduced or learned by the public, they embrace these well, as they understand that toxins are not supposed to stay in our bodies too long. When the detoxification process objectively and subjectively improves their health they begin to build their trust in the nontoxic alternative care recommendations endorsed by Integrative Medicine specialists. We as responsible citizens must be in charge of our own environmental cleanup. And all the synthetic mix of medications or vitamins will not address the underlying cause of own symptoms unless we try to get rid of the cause.

The latest issue that hit our news on this topic is xenobiotics. Xeno means stranger. It is an inorganic chemical that disturbs the hormonal or endocrine system, immune system, and nervous system. This pollutant can damage our DNA and cause gene instability. All of these can predispose patients to cancer and significantly influence the aging process.

Chemicals that disrupt endocrine systems are: DES (Diethylstilbestrol), styrene parathion, mercury, lindane, dioxins, atrazine, chlordane, lead, malathion, and parathion.

There are toxins from our own body called endotoxins. These are intestinal bacteria, fungi, and virus parasites. These can cause poor health and remain as free radicals or living viruses but dormant. An example is the chicken pox virus that is always dormant in our nerve bundle system, and it can return when our immunity is low with a herpes zoster, or shingles, attack.

We all know our bodies are designed to manage internal detox, which is removal of the toxin, viral, or bacterial. Due to an external insult, the immune system is disrupted and low in functioning and is when this detoxification process is not functioning fully or normally. Then we accumulate these toxins, and we need a special detox. The majority of detox occurs in the digestive tract. Our gastrointestinal tract consists of the stomach all the way to the small intestine and large intestine that we call the colon.

Most of the end waste products stay in our colon, waiting for evacuation. Most of nutrition is absorbed through the small intestine (ileum and jejunum). Skin is the largest detox organ and the largest organ period. Through sweating and excretions of the lymphatic and sweat glands, some toxins are excreted. Seventy percent of detoxification takes place in our liver. This is actually called Phase 2 detox.

The detoxification process is impaired during aging. In the elderly with lack of water intake, the detoxification process is also affected. Impairment also reduces absorption of the nutrients from the food we eat. So all of this may disrupt the normal detoxification process. And when this happens, it creates a buildup of toxins and predisposes people to easily getting sick as the immune system will be exhausted. When this happens, the individual gets sick, and this accelerates the aging process.

When we are sick and bacterial infection is the cause, it is common that the conventional medical doctors prescribe pharmaceuticals and antibiotics. The antibiotics disrupt the detoxification enzymes and often kill the probiotics in our digestive systems. Most people do not know that drugs can inhibit the internal inhibition in the liver. Those include drugs like antibiotics, antidepressants, H2-blockers, antiviral medications (Valtrex, Zulvirax, etc.). These drugs can interact and cause an accumulation of a greater inner inhibition of the detox process.

In our practice, we are helping our patients to eliminate pharmaceutical drugs as much as possible and replace them with a similar effect of a nontoxic nutraceutical. That way they recover from the side effects of the drugs, and we slowly restore the function of their natural detoxification process.

Often we have to test the gastrointestinal mucosal lining using a blood and urine test. This way we will rule out leaky gut syndrome and also sensitivity to other material such as gluten and environmental toxins. Often patients misunderstand the reaction of a leaky gut. They always think if they have that condition then they must have diarrhea or severe bowel movement problems. However, leaky gut can be just a delayed reaction to a certain inflammatory food that is not agreeing with our systems at that stage. This situation often is caused by the thinning of the mucosal membrane.

The goal of detoxification is:

1. To reduce the burden of your body's natural detoxification system.

- Reduce the toxic burden by removing the offending toxin, stress, and only take the most necessary drugs.
- Reduce exposure by eating more organic vegetables and meats. Avoid fish that accumulates high mercury, such as tuna.
- Drink plenty of good, purified mineral water.
- Gradually one must review their diet and adjust according to the blood tests that are supporting objective medicine.
- Stop smoking, and taking cannabis and alcohol.
- Abide by the anti-aging diet. Everyone should avoid refined sugar as it causes internal fermentation and increases production of yeast. Also avoid coffee, alcohol, commercially prepared sugar water or juices, sweetened cereals, and caffeinated tea.

2. Always leave the intestinal tract clean so it can be healthy and absorb and detox the nutrient or toxin. How do you leave it clean?

- The food goes down the intestinal tract and also some toxins.
- Before it reaches the colon, the detoxification of bacterial toxins are starting, and the mucosal membrane has an internal automatic barrier so it continues its journey to the large intestine as a final place.
- In this last destination before it is excreted, it is mixed with all kinds of bacteria. Some are called "friendly bacteria," which keeps the balance of the pathogenic ones. They both are anaerobic, which means they can survive without oxygenation.
- Along with them are parasites and yeast, molds, and all kind of salts and digested material, of course.
- There we find the immune substances such as secretory Immunoglobulin A. This protects the neutralization of any foreign substance, and usually this happens before it enters the liver.

- o In our diet, if we eat more fresh fruits and vegetables and fibers and avoid antibiotics that kill these normal microfloras, we supplement with friendly species, and then the detoxification process is easier.
- o When it is unhealthy:
  1. Belly is distended and bloated.
  2. Fatigue and "food coma" syndrome or needing to rest after meals.
  3. Constipation or diarrhea.
  4. Gas and feeling discomfort in the belly after eating or waiting for elimination.
  5. Improve or facilitate the blood and lymphatic natural detoxification system

3. Improve or facilitate the blood and lymphatic natural detoxification system.

    - o During our first evaluation, we always try to include evaluation of toxins in the blood. We need to remove excessive heavy metals, ferritin, arsenic, cadmium, lead, thallium, gadolinium, and so forth. They can inhibit the cell from absorption of nutrients.
    - o The symptoms of toxic blood includes sensitivity to all supplements or drugs, adverse reaction to caffeine, or having so many problems with skin blemishes like pimples, boils and infected hair follicles, and welts.
    - o There is no conventional way to detox your blood, as the doctors are not trained to detect or evaluate these conditions. But many ingredients like echinacea, red clover, and essiac tea protocols, or even the heavy metal binders like Clinoptilolite or the basic compound Na2K-EDTA can be used to detox.
    - o Some people do the fasting method with high temperature heat spa or steam and drink plenty of mineral water. The filtered water leaves the calcium, magnesium, potassium, chloride but removes heavy metals, chlorine and lead in that way.

4. Improve Liver Detoxification Pathway (Detox Phase 2).

    o Looking at the function of the liver. It is very sad to see how people abuse themselves with alcohol intake or acidic drinks like caffeinated coffee or tea, sodas, and eating carbohydrates late at night that cause the liver to work all night long. Having high sugar or fat intake can become addicting.
    o The liver assists carbohydrate, fat, and protein metabolism and breaks them down to a smaller particles so we can use them to produce proper energy according to "Krebs cycle" biology.
    o Your liver also maintains the sugar level. If it fails to do so then you develop an insulin resistant situation where the sugar cannot be metabolized and kept properly. The sugar then goes straight down to the liver and is converted to fat. Then you accumulate fat storage.
    o This big organ actually takes care of filtration of bacteria and is metabolically active to provide energy and carry out the tissue toxins and create tissue renewal.

When your liver is not functioning well:

1. You can have digestive issues, heartburn, floating stool or constipation, and intolerance of alcohol. Then if exhausted, your tongue and skin or sclera is yellowish due to the increase of the bilirubin that can't be metabolized.

2. Skin problems also worsen: acne, rosacea, poor skin tone, brown spots or "liver spots," and spider nevus, or lumps everywhere that has fat in it called cellulite. Likewise nonalcoholic fatty liver disease can develop. You accumulate fat even though you are not an alcohol drinker. Alcohol turns into sugar, and it is the sugar that goes straight to the liver and becomes fat there.

Pillars of Healthy Aging

3. Hormone imbalance syndrome where you have pain during one's period or severe reaction to hormone replacement.

4. Difficulties tolerating the fat-soluble vitamins like Vitamins A, D, E, and K. The skin becomes yellow and sclera turns yellow when given a normal amount of these vitamins.

5. Irritable personality, headache, insomnia, depression and poor concentration. These people feel heat in the upper body or face.

6. Immune system is impaired with allergy symptoms, and chronic fatigue fibromyalgia and systemic infection happen easily, and there can also be viral infection such as hepatitis.

7. When it gets worse, then the face appears yellow and also cellulite is apparent in the skin area.

Products used to detoxify include milk thistle, dandelion, lipotropic substance (amino acid and methionine), choline, folic acid, and vitamin B-12. Food detoxicants are beets, radishes, sprouts, dandelion greens, and more green leafy vegetables.

Secondary organs to detoxify are the kidneys, lungs, skin, and also the lymphatic system.

Some of you are able to do all of the above on your own as a home program, but I recommend that you go through the supervised detoxification if you have abnormal symptoms symptoms, plan also to get serious intense detoxification to get well.

LUNGS

The exchange of gases occurs in the lungs, and blood circulates to be cleansed there, so it is full of oxygen and is delivered though the heart to the whole body to be utilized. Due to outside air pollution, the toxins often cause allergy and T=Rhinitis or sinusitis as well. Some people have so much toxin that they develop an asthma situation. This is called an asthma allergy (due to the irritants).

Gargling with sea salt water may heal the mucosal membrane. But some people train themselves in a deep breathing technique originating from Chinese qi gong and yoga practitioners.

There are more sophisticated methods, but any of this will be a waste when people continue to smoke. Avoid indoor air contaminants or outdoor pollutants as much as possible. The highest polluted air level is in the afternoon. Exercising outside during this time on The street is the worse time due to motor exhaust. Solar radiation also is the highest in the afternoon. Thus morning exercise is best.

SKIN

Toxins are eliminated in the sweat and oils from the sweat glands. Taking a hot bath in Epsom salts or sea salt water is the best and, if done daily, is an excellent routine.

Hot showers with softened, filtered hard water or mineral water is best. The chlorine and other hard minerals will pollute the water that we need for good skin.

Some Koreans and Japanese do dry skin brushing and stay in the sauna. They usually also soak in hot mineral water. It is one of their good hygiene habits.

KIDNEYS

Healthy urine, which is the detox material from our kidney, can be observed as pale yellow without smell. Our urine contains urobilirubin that gives the yellow color. It has no smell until it is oxidized or mixes with the water where the oxygen carried by the water molecule oxidizes it and gives it a smell. Healthy urine does not smell foul. If you are dehydrated, your urine will have a strong odor and be dark yellow in color.

Your kidney is very important as it eliminates toxins from the blood. So when your kidney is not functioning, we often have to dialyze your blood to reduce the accumulation of the toxins that circulate and might kill the person or blind them. Fortunately we have two kidneys, but often it does not show any abnormal blood value of urea or creatinine until both are affected. One usually compensates the other.

Often calcium accumulates and forms a stone due to too much in the diet or due to an abnormal metabolism. This can clog the kidneys from the important function of filtration.

There are several detoxifications that we can practice ourselves at home and also can have that service, as it needs supervision. Either way, you need to make sure that you get evaluated for toxins in the blood. Once you know your status of toxicity then I usually sit with my patients and explain to them where the situation needs some attention. I arrange either the home or the supervised detoxification services that we offer at our facility.

The home detoxification

1. Skin Detox Bath:

    a. Put 1–2 cups full of Epsom salt or pink salt and half full water in the tub. Soak yourself for at least 20–30 minutes

    b. Add 1 quart of 3 percent H_2O_2 or hydrogen peroxide available over the counter, and add 2 teaspoons of sea salt. Soak for 20–30 min or longer.

    c. Skin brushing/scrubs: use a dry loofa sponge (available in the market) and use it to scrub your entire body gently using some natural soap in the warm bathtub. You can do this two or three times a week depending how your skin exfoliates.

    d. Herbal bath tub (used by Chinese or Asians as feet detox), but you can use essential oil and a mix of dry rose petals, lavender flower drops, and or thyme. Drop in a warm tub full of water and soak your body for 20–30 minutes.

2. Connective tissue detoxification (muscles, joints, and ligaments, fats)

    Exercises can do this And cardio like fast walking or slow smooth muscle stretching (yoga, Pilates and Tai-chi). The idea is to improve blood and lymphatic circulation.

    Some massages are for lymphatic drainage enhancement.

    Take extra enzymes systemically; take them in between meals so it is not near digestion to help systemic healing.

    Some people use homeophatic medicine and in my practice we encourage all of the above, including the supervised ones. We use homotoxicology which removes of toxins we use other ingredients that are not toxic to bind the toxin we use chelation and mix together is addressed as a "cocktail".

3. Gastroenterology system or the Colon system.

    Using a home Device as enemas, we can also cleanse our colon. Many people have adapted this "do it yourself" technique and replenish the friendly bacteria by taking some probiotics after the procedure.

The Supervised Detoxification

For many people, supervised detoxification was not common knowledge until recently. Medical doctors who practice homotoxicology are the ones who practice Integrative Medicine. Most patients learn it when they search for further help, as their conventional therapy is not good enough for them.

Supervised detoxification includes:

1. Personalized nutritional supplements. Objective findings of the need of these supplements are determined by testing blood, urine, hair, or saliva specimens.

    Many laboratories support this testing, and physicians undergo special training to understand what to order and how to translate the results.

    It can be very overwhelming for new patients because the result usually is positive, as we know that our world is very toxic. However, this is necessary so we have to be careful not to overtreat. Some patients have been some patients have been getting treated for sometimes. We must be careful not to overprescribe treatments.

We encourage

Preparation by using a special diet of organic fresh fruits and vegetables. It is best to be gluten free during the detoxification period for one day prior and one day after.

Drink enough water and also green drinks that support alkalinity of the body.

Food that supports liver detox are good such as dandelion roots, radishes, chlorella, green vegetables, celeries, wheat grass, and spirulina.

Drinking enough water also promotes detoxification through the kidney and toxin removal through the urine.

There are vegetables that promote urination or work as a natural diuretic. These include parsley, peaches, celeries, peach leaf tea, green leaf tea, and of course pure water.

You need at least 8–10 glasses of water a day. If you are more than 120–120 pounds, then use half of your body weight as the approximate volume of water in ounces per day as your requirement. For example a 200 lbs man would assume 100 ounces of water per day.

If you can't drink that much, I encourage you to train yourself to drink as much by increasing the amount each month. Add cups to the total cups you already have been taking.

Always drink all the water you need in the morning and during the day until 6:00 PM. No more liquid after dinner as we are going to train our bladder not to wake us up at night during our resting period.

It is very important that your body stays asleep during the organ detoxification. That is from 11:00 PM to 4:00 AM. That is the time of morning when many of the gravity or post detox bowel movements happen.

Other herbals that support urination include:

1. Urva ursi (Arctostaphyos)

2. Stinging nettle (Urtica Dioica)

3. Green tea (the real green leaf tea contains no caffeine). It is the only kind of tea that is not fermented. It is very good for combating cancer.

   You need to take it in a high dose, which is why there is a tea-polyphenol study that shows it represents 20 cups of green tea. We recommend 2–3 tablets (in a tablet form) per day, meaning 40–60 cups of green tea per day. No one can drink that much tea every day, but he or she is able to swallow just 1 small tablet three times a day for treatment.

4. Cleavers (Gallium Apatine)

Some doctors and nutritionists would list allowed food during supervised detoxification, but I encourage my patients to do an intense two-week phase 2 (liver) detox every three months. This way, the change of lifestyle is tolerable.

Once they feel better, they adapt slowly to a healthy and recommended diet.

Most of the healthy diets that encourage detox include:

- Small amounts of carbohydrates from organic rice. Quinoa is a better substitute here for rice grains.

- Vegetable: green leafy vegetable lettuces and spinach, kale, bok choy, broccoli, green mustard, radishes, cucumber, onions, green onions, leeks, garlic, and asparagus, and so forth.

    Other vegetables can be eaten if they are on the list of noninflammatory food as demonstrated on their blood test.

- Fruits: low glycemic organic fruit. That does not include grapefruit that inhibits liver detox. Due to the natural sugar content, they are lower in minerals and vitamins compared to vegetables. Limit them in your diet due to the higher glycemic index, as sugar is sugar. Limit your intake of high glycemic index fruits.

- Oils. This is an area where we need to be careful. There are many oils being advertised, such as cold-pressed olive oils as a good essential fatty acid, but they have too much arachidonic acid, which promotes joint inflammation.

- Evening prime rose is the only oil that has no scientific value, but it is found to be very good for hydration and lubrication of synovial fluid and also hormone balancing.

- Flaxseed oil is among the good ones if used carefully. Avocado oils and sunflower seeds oil are also allowed.

- Seaweed is rich in iodine and minerals; it is good for hormone balancing.

- Naturally fermented soy and tamarind (wheat-free soy) is allowed. Bragg's Liquid Aminos and culinary spices that are noninflammatory in the blood tests are good to have.

- Tea or herbal flower tea (chamomile, raspberry, passionfruit, mint, chrysanthemum, jasmine are good because they do not have caffeine.

- Spring mineral water is excellent, and distilled water is also used for detoxification.

- Legumes soy products limited to miso, tempeh, and tofu (nonwheat ones) and bean sprouts.

Nutraceutical for detoxification

In my practice there is no one-size-fits-all Nutraceutical for everyone. After careful examination and evaluation of all results, we usually come up with what needs to be compounded for the patients. The doses match the severity of the degree of risk in the test results. This way when we repeat the test, on the spot check, we will focus on the improvement to optimal value.

Supplements for detoxification are on this list. Most of these are taken in between meals and in two divided doses.

- Antioxidants A, C, E, and selenium in a non-GMO form of its active ingredient and also with the most bioavailability of each.
- All the vitamin B complex according to the doses you need.

- Folic acid or methylated folate if you have a methylation problem. Methyl folate 1 mg, but other forms might require up to 5–20 mg/day
- Selenium 400–1000 mcg/day in divided doses.
- Zinc
- Alpha lipoic acid 300–600 mg in divided doses best with meals
- N acetyl choline 1500–2000 mg /day
- Quinone 300 mg twice/day
- Acetyl L carnitine 1000 mg/day
- L glycine 1000–3000 mg/day
- Probiotic 20–40 billion/day

Other homeopathic remedies

- MSM 500–2000 mg day
- Niacin flush 500–1000 mg/day
- Magnesium: calcium (2:1 ratio) 600–800 mg/day: 400–500 mg/day). Calcium D glucanate is best, and magnesium in glysinate or malate or stearate form can be taken
- Taurine 500–1000 mg/day
- Methionine 1000–1500 mg/day
- Choline 1000–2000 mg/day

I encourage people to do this for two straight weeks every quarter. They can also do this three days every month.

During the detoxification process, patients might experience a detox crisis where toxins are removed in a large amount. They might experience weakness, tiredness, extreme fatigue, need more sleep, or dizziness, which usually last for a few hours or a day.

Some claim a foul smell of their stool or urine. Many notice a body odor change during detoxification.

HYDROCOLONIC

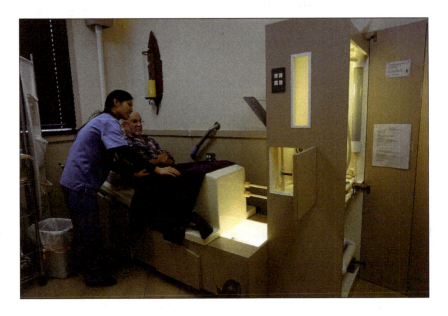

There are many people who do this at home by using a ready-mixed material like coffee enemas, and so forth. The one I have been endorsing for thirty years is called an open system hydrocolonic. In the open system hydrocolonic, the colon is undergoing a cleansing procedure using a small sterile nozzle. The water pressure is about 1 pound. Compare that to 16–20 pounds of pressure in the regular faucet.

Patients come to the office without food for two to three hours or, if they eat, they eat very light and avoid gassy leafy vegetables like broccoli and cabbage.

In the reclining position, the patient usually becomes an expert in no time to operating the "on and off" button and experience some mild peristaltic cramping. Peristalsis is what I call "the exercise of the wall of the colon."

This process of cleansing is under our supervision. After a while, the patients can purchase their own equipment and do it at home should they wish. The evacuation of the colon reaches a peak when it washes the caecum content. Each time we hydrate them. The chance of returning more of the gastrocolonic reflex is better. Most patients are happy to go into maintenance after their first series of three hydrocolonics.

We might be able to solve the mystery of their constipation by observing the content of their cecum or colon when it comes out. This is highly recommended for people who do not have gastro-colonic reflex and are constipated.

INTRAVENOUS DETOX

Everyone knows about this terminology because this has been used since the World War II to the present. Lead poisoning was profound then due to all the postwar rebuilding. People were still not aware of the lead content in the paint.

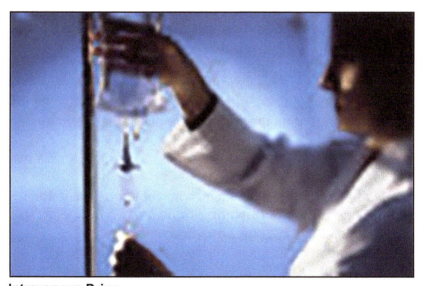
Intravenous Drips

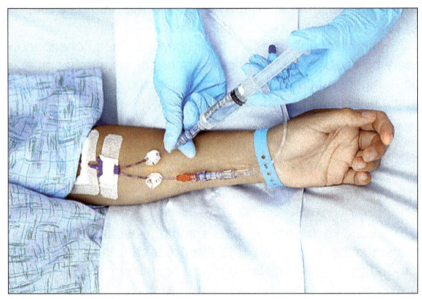

Intravenous Push

This procedure is used for direct absorption into the cells. Most people would prefer not to have it done unless oral treatments alone are not enough.

Some patients are so toxic that oral supplementation will not give a quick success when they are very sick. There are many benefits of intravenous therapy besides being fast and systemic.

1. More concentration of nutritional material can be added without hesitation.
2. Patients might experience more rapid positive effects.
3. Fluids can cross the blood-brain barrier where some oral agents can barely be absorbed.
4. For detoxification, it is the best and the fastest.
5. If done properly, it rarely causes any complications.

Some of the challenges are:

1. The patient has small and brittle veins due to a faster aging process.

2. If they have a problem with drainage and retaining water, then this will involve more fluid.
3. It is more expensive than taking oral supplements. It is not easy to be done in children when a needle is involved.

****

"Let me try a little harder;
Let me pray a little more;
Let me go a little farther
Than I've ever gone before."

—Receive of health

Pillar II
DIET AND NUTRITION

Glycemic Index Table

This next table is taken from the Berkeley Heart Labs, which provides labs that follow the latest Cardiovascular testing, we do this in our office for our patients to ensure their comprehensive chemistry reflects the latest scientific-based evidence for healthy aging. We use IET, International Engineering and Technology Research Scientist NASA, **Ames** Research Center (IET, Ames), also to treat acute and chronic conditions.

The Glycemic Index is a numerical index that ranks carbohydrates based on their rate of glycemic response (i.e., their conversion to glucose within the human body). The Glycemic Index uses a scale of 0 to 100, with higher values given to foods that cause the most rapid rise in blood sugar. Pure glucose serves as a reference point, and is given a Glycemic Index (GI) of 100.

Glycemic Index values are determined experimentally by feeding human test subjects a fixed portion of the food (after an overnight fast), and subsequently extracting and measuring samples of their blood at specific intervals of time.

Glycemic Index
CardioProtective Lifestyle Program

The Glycemic Index (GI) is a measure of how much your blood sugar level rises after a food is ingested. High GI foods cause blood sugar to rise quickly, whereas a food with a low GI causes a smaller rise in blood sugar and may help control established diabetes, aid in weight loss, and lower cholesterol.

Grain/Starch	Grain/Starch	Vegetable	Fruit	Dairy	Protein	Sweets
LOW	**MODERATE (cont.)**	**LOW**	**LOW**	**LOW**	**LOW**	**LOW**
Rice bran 27	Oat kernel bread 93	Peas, dried 32	Cherries 32	Yogurt, low fat, artificially	Peanuts 21	Fructose 31
Barley, pearled 36	Kellogg's Couscous 93	Tomato soup 54	Grapefruit 36	sweetened 20	Beans, dried, not specified 40	Strawberry jam 51
Spaghetti, protein enriched 38	High Fibre Rye Crisp 93	Marrowfat, dried 56	Apricots, dried 44	Milk, chocolate, artificially	Lentils, not specified 41	Cake, sponge 66
Fettuccine 46	Nutri-grain 94	Peas, green 68	Pear, fresh 53	sweetened 34	Kidney beans 41	Ice cream, low fat 71
Spaghetti, wholemeal 53	Life 94	Carrots 70	Apple 54	Milk, regular 39	Butter beans 43	Cake, pound 77
Fruit 'n Oats 55		Yam 73	Plum 55	Soy milk 43	Split peas, yellow, boiled 45	Oatmeal cookies 79
Spaghetti, white 59	**HIGH**	Sweet potato 77	Peach, fresh 60	Milk, skim/nonfat 46	Lima beans, baby, frozen 46	**MODERATE**
Wheat kernels 59	Barley flour bread 95	Sweet corn 78	Orange 63	Yogurt, low fat, fruit sugar sweet 47	Chick peas (garbanzo beans) 47	High Fructose Power Bar 81
All-bran 60	Gnocchi 95	Potato, white, boiled 81	Grapes 66	Milk, chocolate, sugar sweetened 49	Navy beans 54	Pastry 84
Macaroni 64	Grapenuts 96	Potato, new 81	Peach, canned 67		Pinto beans 55	Muesli Bars 87
Linguine 65	Stoned Wheat Thins 96	**MODERATE**	Kiwifruit 75	**MODERATE**	Black-eyed beans 59	Ice cream 87
Rye Kernel bread 66	Wheat bread 97	Beets 91	Banana 77	Ice cream, low fat 71	Chick peas, canned 60	Muffins 88
Instant noodles 67	Taco shells 97	Potato, canned 97	**MODERATE**	**HIGH**	Lentil soup, canned 63	Sucrose (table sugar) 89
Oat bran bread 68	Cornmeal 98	**HIGH**	Fruit cocktail 79	Ice cream 87	Pinto beans, canned 64	Corn Syrup 90
Bulgur 68	Shredded Wheat 99	Potato, mashed 100	Mango 80		Baked beans, canned 69	Shortbread 91
Mixed grain bread 69	Cream of Wheat 100	Rutabaga 103	Apricots, fresh 82		Kidney beans, canned 74	**HIGH**
Pumpernickel bread 71	White bread 100	Pumpkin 107	Raisins 91		Lentils, canned 74	Cake, angel food 95
Bran Buds 77	Golden Grahams 102	French fries 107	Cantaloupe 93			Croissant 96
Special K 77	Water Crackers 102	Potato, microwaved 117	Pineapple 94		**MODERATE**	Corn chips 105
Oat Bran 78	Bagel, white 103	Potato, instant 118	**HIGH**		Split pea soup 86	Graham Wafers 106
Popcorn 79	Kaiser roll 104	Potato, baked 121	Watermelon 103		Black bean soup 92	Donut 108
Rice, brown 79	Bread stuffing 106	Parsnips 139	Dates 141		Green pea soup, canned 94	Waffles 109
Muesli 80	Cheerios 106					Vanilla Wafers 110
	Total 109					Tapioca, boiled with milk 115
MODERATE	Breakfast bar 109					Pretzels 116
Pita bread, white 82	Rice Cakes 110					Honey 126
Bran Chex 83	Post Flakes 114					Glucose 138
Rice, white 83	Rice Krispies 117					Maltose 152
Hamburger bun 87	Cornflakes 119					Tofu frozen dessert, non-dairy 164
Oatmeal 87	Rice Chex 127					
Rye flour bread 92	Rice, instant 128					
	French baguette 136					

Berkeley HeartLab, Inc.
4myheart Center

1 (800) Heart-89 • 1 (800) 432-7889

© 2006 Berkeley HeartLab, Inc.

The earliest known work on the Glycemic Index was done by Dr. David Jenkins and associates at St. Michael's Hospital in Toronto, Canada. More recently, an effort to expand the Glycemic Index has been made by Jennie Brand-Miller and her associates at the Human Nutrition Unit of the University of Sydney in Sydney, Australia.

The Glycemic Index yields some surprises. Nutritionists used to believe that all simple sugars digest quickly and cause a rapid rise in blood sugar, and that the opposite was true for "complex carbohydrates." But that's not always the case. While many sweet and sugary foods do have high GIs, some starchy foods like potatoes or white bread score even higher than honey or table sugar (sucrose)!

INSULIN FACTORS

Have you heard of the "insulin resistance condition"? If you are found to have insulin resistance, you need to remedy it as soon as possible because it leads to many other health problems and major health issues. The good news is you can reset this hormone to a proper level by modifying your lifestyle, with diet and natural medicine and exercise.

Common factors in the clinical aging stage (age 40–60 years old):

1. Eating dinner after 6–7 PM, when the insulin level should be at the lowest level.
2. Carrying a little extra fat due to weight gain. Lack of exercise or hormonal imbalance.
3. Mildly irregular blood pressure or high blood pressure that is difficult to lower without any prescription medication
4. Having a regular annual physical that includes a standard blood test, but not showing if you are insulin if you are insulin resistant or not.
5. Slightly low HDL and slightly higher LDL with lightly high triglycerides without changing our diet for years.
6. Unexplained mood changes, anxiety, and depression.

7. Menopausal syndrome affecting your health.

If you have high blood pressure at this age, most likely you also have insulin resistance.

If you have high blood pressure and insulin resistance and high cholesterol, most likely you will develop a condition called "Syndrome X." Many in this group will also have a pre-diabetic situation or perhaps diabetes.

This triad can lead to serious cardiovascular disease.

Syndrome X findings

1. Type 2 diabetes, insulin resistance, sugar intolerance

2. Cardiovascular hypertension and Low HDL with high triglycerides

3. Elevated uric acid and leptin

4. Overweight and abdominal obesity

INSULIN = AGING MEASUREMENT

You can measure this hormone level by doing blood serum after fasting overnight. This is an easy and faster way to set the pace of your aging.

If you want to measure your gland products of the Human Growth Hormone, or it is called IgF-1 (Insulin Growth Factor 1), which is what we call the "*youth* hormone." This is also the way to do it. It is not easy economically to improve the level.

Growth Hormone is only available through an injection as the molecule is very large (191 amino acids in 1 molecule) so it cannot be absorbed if it comes in any other form. Although through the years, instead of the human source (cadaver in prior to the 1970), now it can be made using a DNA recombinant bacteria or E. coli (Humatrope or Genotropin) and mammal (whale) such as Saizen.

Back to insulin, this should be routinely checked in one's annual physical lab test. But it is very rare that your primary care physician does this test. This is because it was not until recently that anti-aging medicine has linked metabolic disease to diet, lifestyle and nutrition, or hormone balancing in our area, which is Integrative Medicine.

I hope, after reading this book, you will pay a little more attention to the use or function of insulin and the role it has in the annual physical examination and blood test.

The main function of insulin is to:

1. Regulate sugar in our metabolic system thus converting glucose to fat, and glucose to glycogen.
2. It helps break the fat to adipose cells. Regulates the fatty acid (free fatty acid and essential fatty acid).
3. Stimulates growth.
4. It helps in the uptake of amino acids and utilization of protein.
5. Hormone balancing, especially estrogen, which has a role in infertility.
6. It helps in absorption of essential minerals thus maintaining the body's homeostasis.
7. Works in balancing DNA synthesis and cell replication (influences cancer growth) or regeneration from the protein details.

Insulin secretion is proportionate directly to the rise of sugar/glucose. This sugar is related directly to "how many calories you eat."

If your fasting glucose (8–10 hours prior to your blood draw), is above the 90 mg/dl, more insulin is being produced. Insulin will not be needed otherwise.

If this happens consistently, the insulin will rise all the time during the fasting period and eating does not matter. This is called *insulin resistance* or *glucose imbalance*.

GLUCAGON

Since insulin is used to mediate metabolism or anabolic activities, it also is regulated by hormones such as glucagon, cortisol, human growth hormone, adrenaline, epinephrine, and norepinephrine. Since insulin plays an important role for hormone synthesis, especially estrogen; this will effect premenstrual or menopausal syndrome. At a young age, it influences women's fertility. Some women with a high carb diet can have a problem in ovulation or fertility.

Glucagon can act as a catabolic process, or tearing down, process. This is not glycogen; it is glucagon. Glucagon and insulin have to be balanced. When you eat carbohydrate (even high protein), it leads to rising glucose and insulin and glucagon. People gain weight easily or cannot lose weight properly due to high insulin or insulin resistance. When this happens the imbalance in health or homeostasis occurs and aging is accelerated.

Insulin is considered the aging hormone because it has Insulin Receptors Substrate (IRS), a protein that facilitates insulin signaling to the cells in our bodies how to regulate sugar. All of this was discovered and reported in 2000. Before 2000, insulin checking was not too popular but has been since, especially by integrative practitioners.

The pancreatic cells also release glucagon, which is like insulin. Its function is to increase the level of glucose in the blood by breaking down glycogen (sugar that forms in the liver) into glucose. High protein meals or intake of amino acids also activates secretion of glucagon. If hypoglycemia, or low blood sugar levels, occurs, glucagon is activated. If protein is not consumed in the same amount as sugar then the glucose level might be low, and amino acid will be high. This condition induces the secretion of both glucagon and insulin at the same time. This is often done by those who try to build muscles by eating just high protein.

Hormone signaling proteins include fatty acids, cytokines, TNF Alpha (tumor necrosis factor) and peptide such as leptin which is hormone-like in its function in fat regulation and metabolism.

LEPTIN

This protein is manufactured in fat. Often it is called the fat hormone due to its association with working to counteract the "craving instinct." This will influence the amount we eat as well. It will give us satiety after our meal. According to some research, it may be also be related to longevity or healthy aging. Abnormal leptin can lead you to type 2 diabetes.

Glucose metabolism depends on the signaling between muscle and fat. After a meal, the nutrients are broken down (carbohydrates and sugar), broken down into glucose, and taken up by the liver under the influence of insulin. When they are being used, they enter the general blood circulation for the cells, and these later are stored in the liver or used by the muscles and stored as glycogen. Some of this is converted to triglycerides and stored as fat in adipose cells (adipocytes).

TYPE 1 DIABETES

Type 1 diabetes is associated with the failure of the pancreatic islet cells to produce enough insulin. The high glucose and insulin levels cause muscle weakness.

NUTRITION

It would be nice if we did not need to take any supplements, and our bodies could get the necessary nutrition from our diet. Is that possible is the question?

In my practice, we do not second guess in our practice. Those who come to us usually have been attended by conventional doctors and feel worse afterward. They are not willing to continue in trial and error taking prescription medications for their symptoms such as:

- Low energy
- Can't sleep at night
- Wake up not rested, after sleeping all night

- Cannot stand the side effects after they tried taking prescription drugs.
- Muscles get weaker and tendons are torn after taking an antibiotic, such as Cipro.
- Constipated, even on a veggie diet.
- Feel bloated with lots of gas during the day
- Pain over all the joints, and every doctor has said there was no problem in the examination.
- Scared due to multiple steroid injections and oral steroids.
- Given hormone replacement therapy without checking the blood level.
- Migraines are getting worse.
- Hair is thinning.
- Can't lose weight and keep gaining weight with change of diet.
- Can't stop eating sugary stuff.
- Addicted to coffee and sweets.
- Can't concentrate.
- Short-term memory is fading and find it difficult to recall things.
- Only forty years of age but have no sexual drive, and my doctor said, "Everything is normal."
- Having stress and depression but have problems with anti-depressants from their doctor or can't tolerate them.

On and on, and probably these things are happening to you and you don't know who you should see.

Conventional medical schools offer only four to six hours of nutritional education. Mainly we learned about vitamin A, D, E, and K, when we are low in them, what to do when they are low, and what the symptoms are.

We never learn about which supplement helps to prevent diseases. Additionally, we do not learn what nutrition is needed to improve our memory or perhaps our sleep quality to stop the insomnia. We never learned what kind of test should be conducted when those symptoms occur. All we learned was if we eat three meals a day, that was healthy enough. If we aren't healthy, then take medication like normal people do.

It has been documented in many scientific journals with peer review studies that supplementing your diet (food) with optimum levels of vitamins, minerals, enzymes, probiotics and many other supplements would help our system to detox or function better and help in the healthy aging process. Nutrition is probably one of the fastest growing industries currently competing with the pharmaceutical drugs. The population is pushing the knowledge and technology of nutrition to improve their results in health from its contents.

Not all nutrients give an anti-aging effect where it can actually deter the process of aging. When we use anti-aging supplements, we specifically use it so that it addresses a specific issue and prevents possible deterioration in our living cells that might accelerate the aging process.

Since early 1800 homeopathic medicine was already used in Russia. Since 1500 BC people used blood that has iron to treat dizziness and also blood given in the diet after birth in China. 1900 was when we discovered some vitamins, and since then advanced technology has already improved the quality and absorption of the active ingredients of vitamins. Since 1990 the vitamins, minerals and all other supplements are so improved that the FDA has allowed some of the superior quality ones that have been studied to be categorized as "nutrition that have pharmaceutical effects," since called nutraceuticals. This is to differentiate this type of medicine from the pharmaceutical drugs.

However, we can also find medical health professionals who do not follow the progress of natural medicine or nutraceuticals and tell their patients that they question the efficacy of nutraceuticals.

Like other knowledge, the patients sometimes Google or find the information on the Internet and compare information. However the medical information is often full of medical words and terminology and names that they can't even pronounce. This makes it difficult to access them on the Internet. If they do find them, they are often not interested because the side effects of the drugs would scare them to death.

The progress of nutraceutical education in the community is slow, and patients are not going to wait for their doctors to learn this in their own sweet time. That is, even if the doctors are going to do it because many doctors are too busy to spend time to learn something new. Therefore, these patients seek advice and go to naturopathic physicians who are trained solely in natural medicine and not conventional drugs. Since 1980, medical communities who are open minded and willing to learn and teach the others would gather their friends and form their own associations. The first one is called the Academy of Advancement in Medicine. I was so fortunate to have gone the right direction and learned this from my elders or colleagues that had done so earlier than me. I soon begin to realize that there is resistance by the conventional medical society to this knowledge. It takes about thirty years for some of them to hear about us through their own patients. Many of my patients found me from searching the name of listed physicians at the ACAM.org website.

ACAM is very unique and known for detoxification. Since 1990, dozens of other associations have formed, and the other one that pioneers in balancing hormones is Academy of Anti-Aging Medicine. Dr. Klatz and Glodman, osteopaths, were the visionaries for hormone replacement therapy. The late Dr. John Lee MD was the one who actually started natural progesterone back in 1990, and he is known as one of the fathers of bio-identical hormone replacement therapy. He emphasized use of progesterone as a protective hormone.

Soon after that, another association called International Institute of Functional Medicine was founded by a nonmedical doctor, Dr. Jeffrey Bland, PhD, FACN, FACB, CNS. Dr. Bland was the author of the book called *The Disease Delusion*. In 1990, he was a CEO of Health Com. International, a global company who produced nutritional products. Currently Dr. Bland started the Personalized Lifestyle Medicine Institute (PLMI) in Washington.

From these associations, many of our patients read articles that make more sense to them than reading a leaflet about medication from the pharmacy. That is how they learn that there is hope with a natural sort of nutrition that can help them replenish what substances they lack in their bodies.

Pillars of Healthy Aging

Supplementation of nutraceuticals has become very sophisticated now that it is available through oral tablets, capsules, caplets, powder, liquid, and even in gel form. You can even find injectable forms and suppository forms. Some are in pellet form where it is implanted in your bodies. Then it gives you the medication, using a time-release technology for four to six months at a time.

Important points to remember

1. Never take any supplements unless you need them. Lab chemistry testing can show you the deficiency you have.
2. Use as good a quality supplement as possible because not all supplements are the same. They also vary in the form and delivery system they are bound to.
3. Current doses often need to be repeated, and follow up appointments with your doctor and testing is highly recommended so you don't keep taking unnecessary supplements. In some cases, you may need more of the product. It is just like medication; you need supervision to do it right.
4. The dose also varies with the severity of the condition or the goal for recovery at the time.
5. The source of the ingredient is very important as labeling cannot tell the untrained person to recognized the source. FDA regulations are set, but not all manufacturers follow them.
6. Some vitamins at a certain dose work for a different target organ and treatment. Take vitamin C that is widely used and sold outside. Some people think taking ascorbic acid of 1000 mg is the requirement for health. However some people who have chronic infection would need 3000–5000 mg. Also the Ascorbic Palpitate form is probably safer to take rather than Ascorbic palmitate acid due to the source that is usually corn based and very rarely is organic. Cancer patients may need 25,000—50,000 mg of intravenous vitamin C as it can irritate the stomach if you take it in high doses by mouth.

7. The form matters as the absorption changes from best as liquid to the least, in tablet form, in which you may absorb less than 10 percent.

We do not follow all the RDA that needs to be listed due to the regulations anymore because it is very difficult to set a recommended daily allowance after considering the entire seven situations above.

The initial RDA was set to prevent common diseases for average people as scurvy, gum disease, or dry skin. But that also depends on your age. If you are young enough, say under forty, are in good health, have no problems with stress or being overweight, or have any conditions like a toxic liver, and not taking medications, then your health may alter the efficacy of vitamins.

I hope you understand what nutrition means. What we need to focus on now is the practical way of taking nutrition.

UNSUPERVISED

1. If you are at least twenty-five years of age and maintain a good diet, do not get sick easily, are a nonsmoker, a nondrinker, and exercise two hours minimum a week, Then you simply need a basic multivitamin with good calcium (800 mg), magnesium (800 mg), and vitamin D3 (2000 IU) with minerals and digestive enzymes.

   You notice the Cal:Mag ratio is 1:1. Calcium versus magnesium is required. This is to bring the calcium to the bone. Vitamin D3 is required also because it is responsible to glue calcium down to the bone so it is not traveling unattended in our blood. The purpose of this is so the calcium does not lodge in the blood or sticky places along the arteries or in the joints then create a spur or bone spur ten to twenty years later. Vit D3 is vital with calcium mineral supplements.

   It is very important to avoid the tablet form of calcium. Capsule form and vegetarian capsules is probably the best.

2. If you are younger than twenty, most likely you are still eating at home with healthier food being served as well and may need fewer vitamins. This is assuming you are eating nutritious organic food at home. But if you are not, then you need to take the amount specified above. Children less than eight years old should take half of the above level of vitamin D 3.

3. If you are ages twenty-five to forty, you can certainly add more vitamin D3 up to 3000 IU. If you are bearing a child, then you need a prenatal formula with a higher dose of calcium, like 1500 mg, and obviously you can hardly match the magnesium unless your digestive system allows you to absorb it. A good blood test by your integrative doctor will tell you.

   Otherwise magnesium can irritate the stomach, and you may develop diarrhea. This is not a negative side effect, but you do not want to have this reaction when you have a baby in your womb. Magnesium is healthy for both mother and the baby, and it can prevent eclampsia and preeclampsia or high blood pressure during gestational period.

   This science has been established in the OBGYN conventional sciences. Those who are not given enough magnesium and calcium by their doctor should seek some help from other doctors. After all it is your baby, and you want a healthy baby and easy delivery.

4. Doctors can conduct a red cell pack essential element test to check your minerals at true levels. I always do this when my patients are ready to take supplements for a long time. This is good to check so you don't take too many unnecessary supplements. Conventional chemistry panel blood tests during your annual check or physical does not check this. Thus if not supervised, most likely you will miss knowing what level of minerals you may need. Many

doctors do not prescribe the adequeate test to determine your needs.

5. If you are older than forty years old, I would recommend that you check the true level of your minerals at this stage. You are entering a clinical stage of aging, and you need to make sure all the clinical symptoms are addressed. Liquid supplements or powders are a better choice for addressing your needs, as the absorption is better for you.

6. At age 60, doctors usually give some sort of medication or another. This is the age group that should not stay unsupervised.

SUPERVISED

1. Patients of all ages can be tested using a standard proper nutritional evaluation. We can measure all vitamins, minerals, amino acids, essential fatty acids, and hormones. All biological markers would certainly help us to measure your biological age, and we compare that to your physiological age.

2. Absorption ability and organ functions are aging, as well. This can also be measured, using a blood test. We would also determine your genetic issues. Good use of these numbers helps us explain the cause of the small percent of genetic diseases.

3. In certain blood results, we can see the optimum value and what supplements are needed.

OPTIMUM VALUE

This is taken from the average healthy American. If your value falls in this category, then you are among the average 50 percent of healthy Americans. If you come to my office with some symptoms, you know why the optimum stage is not always what we call healthy because "average healthy Americans" are not always as healthy as they appear. Often they are wondering who they should see or what they should eat or take to improve their health.

This can be improved to a wellness stage and then the healthy aging stage. The later stages of life are when you should depend on the lab results, and you need someone to tell you how much supplementation you need to take. We can tell if you taking too much or not enough, depending on your blood or other tests. Then it is important to compare that result with your next tests to see your progress toward healthy aging.

THE INTERMEDIATE RISK GROUP

If your value falls here, that means your health carries the risk of getting a disease, and 60 percent of the average healthy aging American are healthier than you. The 50 percent is the optimum stage and is definitely where you want to be. Normally the intermediate stage is a warning stage as it can fall to the next less healthy one called the:

HIGH-RISK GROUP

In my office and if you use our contracted lab, then you can see that this is colored as red on your test results. No one likes to see this red color. Psychologically, the patients are affected, and you can see that they are disappointed. This stage means 80 percent of the average healthy American population is healthier than you.

You can tell that this group is at risk and can result in unpleasant health and could deteriorate to where they need some nutrition medication, though it might not be fast enough to help them. Many patients came into my office in this stage, and they find out if they do supplement their diet with nutraceuticals, they can reverse this high risk to intermediate and even optimum health. If they do not them, there might be serious consequences.

I check the chemistry for cardiovascular health, their immune system, and the condition of formation of early plaque. Sometimes their situation might require us to use conventional treatment or send them for further consultation. We make sure that they understand that a conventional doctor might want them to be treated only with drugs.

However, I am very impressed by all my patients who usually are so well informed in the negative effects of such treatments. They follow our instructions and usually improve within four or five months. When they see improvement in their next chemistry check is when our trust is built. Then they stay with the natural products. From there, it is our mutual teamwork that takes them slowly to healthy aging, greater longevity, and active healthy aging levels.

The reason why we deteriorate is when we are aging, the body runs out of steam and we lack the energy or the ability to stay active. Also our digestive system may not be functioning at optimum levels. The production of hormones and enzymes also slows down. This situation is setting you up for health problems that start with these symptoms. However, we find that these symptoms can be corrected by adding the missing nutrients.

By definition, growing old is a deficiency in nutrients. But in the past this deficiency was filled by drugs or ignored by conventional doctors. Some patients said that they want to grow old gracefully. But does it require suffering? Some conventional doctors would say that pain in the joints is "part of old age," and that it should be "well accepted." I laugh when I see an eighty-year-old patient complaining of imbalance and dizziness, and the conventional doctors would quickly instruct the nurse to check their blood pressure and then flip the chart to check if the patients is in on high blood pressure medication. When he confirms that the blood pressure is fine, usually he would prescribe headache medication, such as Tylenol or something with aspirin, and a walker or a cane. Then he might tell them to be careful as this is part of the normal reaction from the drugs he prescribes and also old age, of course.

What should we do? Well we should interview the patient about their diet the day or two before. Did they drink enough fluid, especially when it is summertime? Do they take their medication on a regular basis? Then we need to consult the latest blood chemistry they have with us. Do they have a lack of minerals or vitamin B? Perhaps they are dehydrated. We offer hydration and also a vitamin boost to see if it makes them feel better. The unbalanced situation they are in is going to require them to return so we can evaluate further for any specific neurological condition like normal pressure hydrocephalous or muscle weakness in the legs. We also want to make sure they do not fall at home. Yes, the cane or walker is appropriate at this age as a precaution.

As they grow older, often they fail to drink water as they should. Very often they are lacking fluid, which can easily cause dizziness or imbalance symptoms. Falls are one important thing for the elderly to avoid. This can cause more problems as almost 80 percent of the population older than 80 have osteoporosis.

The good news is that most patients taking vitamin and minerals for healthy aging are improving and these are safe with no side effects. This alone gives them more security when they do not have to worry about fighting the negative side effects of the drugs.

Most elderly don't even know what the side effects of the drugs are that they already have taken for years; properly prescribed by their physicians. It is our job as health professionals who practice Integrative Medicine to slowly remove those drugs when it is endangering their lives and replace them with safer medications like vitamins and minerals.

MEGA DOSE SUPPLEMENTS

As you probably guessed, a mega dose is the dose that is not recommended by our FDA or RDA or whatever organization. What is it? A mega dose is whatever is exceeding those FDA regulations and RDA standards. There is no benefit in consuming amounts exceeding what you need. However if you are taking mega doses because you need them, then that is what you need to take.

SAFE AND EFFECTIVE

These two words go hand-in-hand with measurement of supplements or vitamins. Since there is no negative side effects if taken properly, then the caution factor is to make sure everything is taken in the right amounts and at the proper intervals.

In my thirty years of practice, I know immunoglobulin reactive action can cause inflammation. I find we can be one step safer by checking the allergic reaction to some of the food as the basis of nutrients as supplements. For example, if someone is tested as severely positive taking curcumin. Then as an anti-inflammatory, I would use a different measure such as MSM or Cats Claw or enzymes like boswelia. This is the safest way.

Although nutrients are generally safe, those who want to start taking their health seriously might want to consult the doctors who are well versed in this field before self-medicating. For those who are taking other drugs, especially blood thinners, Coumadin, statins, antidepressants, and so forth, you must inform your Integrative Physician. They make sure it does not cause an adverse reaction when they take a good amount or mega dose of a supplement.

Even though optimum doses, like I have said, are effective and safe, they might interfere with the efficacy of any hypertension drugs. For example should the blood pressure drop as a result of taking vitamins or supplements, then we need to cut the drugs back and depend on the supplement. Obviously the effectiveness depends on the absorption. This also depends on the intestinal mucosal lining, or membrane, of the patients who take the supplements.

As usual, before any operative procedures, you should safely stop taking all supplements. If necessary, ask your doctors who gave you the supplements, and they can advise which is reactive as a blood thinner. These groups are the only group that might cause unnecessary prolonged bleeding time. These are Omega 3, E, Gingko, CoQ-10, herbals, and enzymes,

I normally personalize the supplement to the patient's need, but an initial trial is required to see how they tolerate my regimens. I might ask them to do a compounding program for between one and four months. It is safer to go slow as some patients come with an extremely low level of nutrients, far from the optimum levels. If you give them too much, then it can confuse the body and it will not get metabolized for the proper use, being wasted in their urine.

That is also why some people in the old days said that taking vitamins is a waste of money but only creates expensive urine. I would agree if you take synthetic-based supplements, but it is different when you take a natural food-based supplement, which is gluten free and GMO free. All of these conditions of quality are possible with the new technology of different delivery systems.

New Developments in Alternative Medicine

The new research, development, and formulations in nutrition therapeutics has given Integrative Medicine physicians better leverage in helping their patients, we use more alternative therapies and less drugs, thus avoiding side effects. We are physicians who integrate as much as possible programs to assure our patients healthy aging using a program that does not inhibit healthy aging.

In my practice, I put together a program that is natural, and it has medicinal effects to help our patient's symptoms. We train our staff in this field because many of the medical assistants, or other estheticians were trained in the conventional ways. We train them to understand the concept of Integrative Medicine and healthy aging. We train them to use the latest technologies and to prepare nutrition plans. Every six to twelve months, we review our preparations to follow the progression of the current technology with their delivery system.

This is very important because I always tell my patients that their decision in embarking into alternative medicine is probably not covered by third-party insurance who think that since these regimens are not "drugs," they will not be covered. However more and more alternative medicine hopefully will be covered. Under the new system called the Affordable Care Act preventive care is often covered now.

Doctors know that this nontoxic program would keep the patients healthier and cut the health cost in the United States or the world. However, since it is an emerging field that is only thirty years old, it may take more time as the leaders in the medical field do not change easily. Since the drug companies have a financial interest in keeping things the way they are, only the patients can apply pressure to change.

We try to support and fully commit to help our patients achieve their health goals, while maintaining safety and effectiveness of the program by not resorting to using drugs unless it is really necessary. We work with the manufacturing companies that are licensed by the US Food and Drug Administration and that follow their labeling system and regulation. However, as we all know when it is a nutraceutical product, we need to list on the bottle that it is *not approved* by the FDA. The FDA regulates that. To differentiate from the *drugs* that are approved by the FDA, with their side effects, all manufacturing companies have to put on these disclaimers when the substance is a nutraceutical.

As a licensed physician, I often prescribe alternative therapies. This is treated as medicine due to its medicinal effects. Therefore the doses are usually based on your health chemistry laboratories results.

SOME NUTRACEUTICAL PRODUCTS

The following medication we use and regularly recommend to our patients.

- **Essential Concentrated Nutrient (ECN)**, a liquid multivitamin that has the best absorption and has the proper natural-based food products for every age. Men and women both can use these products as their foundation of their daily multi-vitamin.

- **Nutraceutical with Energy (Capsule)**

This is an encapsulated multivitamin, it has some ingredients that give a boost of energy.

- **Cardio–complete**

    This compound is for cardiovascular health, including problems with artery insufficiency, conduction impairment, and optimizing mitochondrial functions. It helps reduce the endothelium function and helps alleviate physical stress and emotional stress.

- **Re-Start pack**

    This is for detoxification of the liver, kidney (phase 2 detox). This two-week fasting program is a replacement of two meals, using a high quality of vegetarian protein of 18 grams per serving to maintain muscle while detoxing the liver enzyme system that drives the detoxification process. It also has all the multivitamins required for enzyme support and nutrient balance in phase one and two metabolic pathways.

    This safe system of detoxification is essential and we also include the amino acids to prevent production of intermittent metabolites that could cause symptoms of sensitivity or reactions during the detoxification program.

    Many people want to detox, but they need supervision to understand that doing a proper detoxification protects their metabolic pathways for detoxification. We allow our bodies to restart with good cell function this way.

    I encourage people to do this every three to four months if they live in a metropolitan area, like where I am in Pasadena, California.

- **Green Complete**

  Many aging people do not have the time to create alkaline water, so taking a dark green powder drink would help to alkalinize their body. It is also a high antioxidant and potassium-rich source preparation.

- **Cal-Mag-D (Calcium, Magnesium, and Vitamin D3)**

  This is prepared with a proper ratio for younger ages or aging people to ensure that all calcium is taken with magnesium for the tissues, such as bone. This to prevent forming plaque calcification in our arteries or spur calcification. Many from the old school took only calcium and did not include magnesium of an equal amount or more. That is not wise. Vitamin D is the basis of our anticancer and bone building, as it glues the calcium to the bone.

- **Solufiber**

  These are nutrient-based dense soluble fiber drinks that promote healthy gut and healthy cardiovascular and immune systems. Research studies showed that an average person consumes 12 grams of fiber daily, but the minimum healthy adult needs 25–30 grams a day.

  This fiber mix has both soluble fibers (80 percent) that have a significant health benefit of binding the unnecessary fat and taking it out through the gut system, thus maintaining healthy cholesterol levels.

  The insoluble fibers (20 percent) that are commonly found in the over-the-counter section, that aid gut motility and constipation or movement of waste products in the colon are.

- **Coenzyme Q 10**

    This enzyme improves microcirculation and helps the muscles of the heart and micro circulation of the brain.

    - Quinone
    - Quinol
    - PQQ

    The latter is also called Q enzyme Shi Jajit. This is more effective for memory and cognitive function, as well.

- **B-pep max**

    Elderly people who do not have enough acid to digest their food, experience digestion problems and a bloated feeling after eating. Betaine HCL 1000 mg and pepsin 100 mg (gluten free) are in this compound to help them prepare their digestive enzymes for the meal they eat.

- **Probiotics**

    Probiotics (several kinds), such as Probio 5-AB, Probio 20B, and probios 225B, are some of the most advanced and effective formulations of probiotics on the market. They help to maintain good bacteria in the gut responsible for proper digestion and absorption of nutrients from one's diet. This is also important for skin health. It is helpful for combating candida. It is manufactured in a way that protects its friendly bacteria.

    The amount of good bacteria varies from 5 billion to 225 billion. The quality affects the potency, of course. Each of the bottles were tested to make sure that no bacteria were harmed, and you get the product that has live, viable, biologically active bacteria. Dead bacteria do not do you any good.

- **Reishi**

    High molecular weight reishi mushrooms grown in a non-toxic environment are reported to have an anticarcinogenic effect and drives the ability of cancer or anaerobic cells to self-destruct in a process called *apoptosis*. It enhances the immune system. It contains high glycoprotein and polysaccharides.

    This medicinal mushroom boosts your immune system and increases the number of NK cells (Natural Killer cells). This is an Asian medicine. It is very powerful and extremely rare mushroom that has been successfully used for generations in Asia for various health conditions including: hypertension, liver detoxification, insomnia, gastric ulcers, arthritis, asthma, bronchitis, neuromuscular disorders, and much more. Reishi also can alleviate anxiety and help diminish the sensation of pain.

    The dosage for maintenance of 500–1000 mg/day for healthy aging is recommended and 3000–4000 mg/day for immune-compromised patients.

- **TAURA PURE**

    Taura Pure contains the pharmaceutical grade of taurine. It is a free form of amino acid that participates in an assortment of metabolic processes, including glucose uptake, cell membrane transportation, and sodium, potassium, and magnesium regulation.

    It helps regulate the nervous system. It is a sulfur-containing amino acid, which can be beneficial in fighting irregular heartbeat. It is also used in the liver where it is incorporated into bile acids for reabsorption of fats and lipid soluble vitamins. It also helps when one experiences the depletion of hepatic enzymes. Taurine is found in meats, fish, milk, and eggs but not in vegetable proteins; it is very helpful for vegetarians.

- **Leptica-AF**

    This is to help leptin-resistant people. Leptin is a 167 amino acid polypeptide discovered in 1994. Leptin means "thin" in the Greek language. In fact it helps burn fat in the body. It is to help people stop their craving for sugar and hunger. It manages their appetite and decreases their urge to snack. It enables them to taste food better and stimulates metabolism which complements a weight management program.

    We provide alcohol free (AF) homeopathic leptin, which is safe and nontoxic with no side effects.

    People who are insulin resistant should test their leptin and adiponectin, to see if the hormone that controls their fat is working to break down their fat.

- **Liquid Om-3 and OM3-Plus**

    Omega 3 has many important health benefits including:
    Preventing coronary heart disease
    Keeping blood triglyceride at a good level
    Has an anti-inflammatory property
    Enhances immune system
    Helps regulate diabetic blood sugar
    Helps depression and allergies

    There are many Omega 3s available in the market. But it is important to remember that there are many grades of quality. The purity and the quality is very important and also the quality of the capsules themselves. We use the highest grade where we make sure that this has EPA and DHA from the cold-water fish that is free from mercury properties.

- **Rest Best with ONCO**

    The famous grape seed extract antioxidant Onco once had the most scientific papers written among many other excellent nutraceutical papers. Combining this and baby broccoli seeds (SGS= Glucorhaphine), Sulphoraphane Gluco Sinolate found in 1992 by the John Hopkins scientist (400 studies reported), would make this compound an extra strong antioxidant and reduce free radicals in our oxidative, stress-filled environment. It is in our program of oxidant elimination (Detoxification pathways in the cellular system). This boosts the phase 2 enzyme in detoxification against potential carcinogens, and its antioxidant action can stay in the system for seventy-two hours. This was reported to have a significantly higher antioxidant effect than vitamin C, beta carotene or tocopherol E).

    Our proprietary blend of 1450 mg with some synergistic ingredients is excellent in reducing ferritin, which can block the absorption of good nutrients from the food you eat in your diet.

- **One Flush**

    This contains aloe extract that aids the patients to move their bowel contents when their reflex is low.

- **EZ Sleep**

    Sleep is so important. We recognize that. If you can't sleep, the natural herbals such as phenibut, valerian root,

    5 HTP, L theanine, melatonin, taurine, and passion flower extract would help you reach a good night's sleep. We provides a blend of 1200 mg, and some people need more for a booster dose.

- **C-Factor**

    Vitamin C is the most popular vitamin in the world. There are thousands of vitamin Cs in the market. Many of these pills are made using inexpensive manufacturing methods and are in a tablet form.

    Our C-factors are a special time-released formula that allows the gradual release of the active ingredient over a prolonged period of time to coincide with natural biological absorption processes. This special formula is derived from non-GMO corn, and it is 100 percent digested and absorbed into the body. Bioflavonoids and rose hips, as a mixture, are a natural source of vitamin C that has been added to the ascorbic acid to help release the absorption and utilization of our vitamin C formula.

- **Cholesterol Block**

    If your doctor needs to lower your cholesterol, instead of jumping to statin drugs, I would encourage you to adjust your diet and get some good essential fatty acids. Try Red Yeast Rice; it may surprise you. One of the benefits of these products is they have no side effects to your liver and do not cause fatigue, which is most important.

- **E COMPLETE**

    Vitamin E can help to stop the progression of the aging process. This inhibits the cross link of endogenous proteins, important for the stability of cell membranes.

    Vitamin E is an antioxidant that helps to protect against the toxic effects of many chemicals found in air pollutants, especially ozone and carbon monoxide. They also protect our bodies against toxic metals like leads, arsenic, radium, gadolinium, and mercury.

400 IU 100 percent of mixed tocopherol is recommended because tocopherol was found to be more bio-available than the synthetic vitamin E brands that are available everywhere.

The latest finding is of Gamma and Delta Tecotrienol E from Annatto fruits, that has a higher absorption compare to the regular tocopherol . And it is more popular and recommended to be taken by itself and not as a mix tocopherol.

- **Methyl Folate**

  Since 40 percent of the patients who are taking psychiatric medication have a variant of the coagulation gene, it is worth checking for it. Methylated folate and methyl cobalamin would help their symptoms such as anxiety, stress, depression, psychiatric disorders, attention deficit disorders, and many more conditions of the central nervous system.

  Pharmaceutical companies are also making a high dose of this folate for severely affected patients. The doses would be given according to the severity of the patient's lab findings.

- **Malic Plus**

  Malic Plus is a scientific blend with magnesium and malic acid to provide synergistic support for energy production. It is most critical for the production of (Adenotriphosphate) and has been clinically shown to play an integral role in maintaining muscle comfort.

- **Melatonin 3mg—SR**

  This preparation contains pure pharmaceutical grade melatonin and is manufactured under the strictest General

Manufacturing Practices (GMP) guidelines in precise time-release tablets. It is a hormone produced at night and secreted by the pineal gland (the time keeper of the brain and controller of our circadian rhythms). Melatonin appears to be the hormone that regulates biological rhythms and may keep the body clock in sync.

This can be used for insomnia, difficulties maintaining sleep as this is a SR (slow-release) type and also helps people to recover from ordinary travel or jet lag. Research shows that it also works as a powerful antioxidant and helps cancer prevention.

Recent findings suggest that for aging population, we need about 60 mg melatonin as a supplementation for daily consumption. This is to rebuild the sensitivity of the eyes to darkness thus it helps to sleep better in the dark. To improve immune system and also to improve our brain function and prevent memory lost. This does should be taken early afternoon or before 5:00 pm. For immune compromise, this can be taken up to 240 mg per day.

In a certain countries, many of the patients with cancer situation benefit from taking this high dose Melatonin. The latest of reports during the 12th IOICP (International organization of Integrative Cancer Physicians) in San Diego 2017. I personally benefit from taking the 60 mg daily since. I feel better rested in the early morning when I wake up and sleeping early at 9:00 or 10:00 pm becomes much easier for me.

- **Prostate Formula**

One hundred percent of men will experience prostate enlargement or malignancy in their life. This can be prevented by using a natural blend of organic fruits and plants.

We recommend a compound of saw palmetto, a beta sitosterol plant with pygeum, an enzyme that helps keep a healthy prostate. Patients find it helps to relax some of the muscles and prevent frequent urination or difficulty starting urination. Some men have an issue with sexual performance due to their prostate problems.

- **Menopause Formula—Meno Blend**

This is an effective combination of all natural herbs, which have been scientifically selected and balanced to help normalize hormone levels in women. The goal is to control the unpleasant effects of menopause or pre-menopause. Each herb has been carefully selected based on the latest scientific research.

Soy is a flavone and Black Cohosh has been used for years to relieve menopause symptoms and estrogen activity. Wild Yam is a natural source of progesterone. Dong Quay and Licorice root promote vitality. Only the standardized active forms of each ingredient is used in this formula. This is an important aspect in dealing with herbal formula ensuring the potency and consistency of efficacy.

- **MSM (Methy Sulfonyl Methane)**

MSM is a natural source of sulphur and provides pain relief and anti-inflammatory benefits without side effects unless you are allergic to sulphur, although MSM has a different bonded sulphur. However, I would check it first. It helps maintain the structure of keratin and is essential to hair and nail growth. MSM also aids the protection of immunoglobulin, thus supporting the immune system.

MSM 100 mg of nature-pure methyl sulfonyl methane derives from DMS (dimethyl sulfide) that originates in pine trees. MSM supplies the body with organic sulfur necessary for many metabolic processes crucial to maintaining healthy tissues.

- **NATO-MAX**

    Nattokinase is the latest and most exciting natural compound which comes from the Natto traditional Japanese food form of boiled and fermented soybeans. The Japanese have consumed this natto bean for years and have found that it fosters cardiovascular health. It also works as an enzyme that works as a blood thinner, and some tests shows that it dissolves 50 percent of blood clots in less than two hours. It has now more than twenty-five studies, including human trials. It has fibrinolytic activity properties and dissolves the fibrin in blood clots. It comes in capsules or gel capsules. There are many current studies regarding this compound.

- **Niacinamide**

    This form of vitamin B3, niacinamide, has the property to reduce inflammation, osteoarthritis pain, and helps dementia and also insomnia

- **Niacin**

    Niacin is part of vitamin B3 and plays a role in metabolism of protein, fats, and carbohydrates. It also regulates the synthesis of sex hormones.

- **Nitrous ARG (Nitrous Argenine)**

    This compound contains an effective combination of L-arginine, L-lysine and L-ornithine. It is also a combination of citrus bioflavonoids, and medium-chain triglycerides to help increase nitric oxide synthesis.

In 1998, the Noble prize was awarded to three American scientists for the discovery of these nitric oxides, which are biologically active molecules important to healthy aging. Nitric oxide is naturally produced in the body from L-Arginine. Nitrous ARG can help promote healthy blood pressure and improve cognitive function.

- **Leci-pure**

This is an all-natural supplement needed by your brain and every cell in your body. Lecithin is a fat like substance that is produced on a daily basis by the liver and is needed by every cell in your body. Lecithin is an integral nutrient for cell membrane integrity. It helps facilitate the movement of fats from the cells. It is also been found to help improve cardiovascular health. This is a non-GMO soy in a highly absorbable and bioavailable soft gel form, making it easier to take.

- **Lycell–DS**

This takes L-lysine to the next level of cardiovascular support. It is made of 100 percent pharmaceutical grade of L-lysine HCl. Research has shown that L-lysine helps decrease the risk of cardiovascular disease and stroke. It also helps to improve the mucosal membrane and the wall integrity of the vascular walls.

- **Pregnenolone SR**

It is a 100 percent pure pregnenalone, and is pharmaceutical grade. It serves as a precursor of progesterone, a sex hormone. It is known as the "mother of all hormones." That means the entire steroid hormone derives from pregnenolone.

Some of these products cannot be sold over the counter to those under eighteen years old of age unless it is recommended by their physician for some special cases of hormone imbalance.

- **ZINC**

Elemental chelated zinc. Using a glucometer to check your sugar levels and proteinase is important for absorption and utilization in the body.

There are many more super-food nutraceutical products, but the most important thing is this: to replenish what your body needs. It is important not to overlap in products. That is a waste of money, and it can get expensive. It is important to detect any overlap in products for health reasons, also. Not all products are the same as they come with a different concentration and different packages (gluten free, GMO free or a vegetarian capsule which is better than gelatin). The best is liquid preparation, but it costs more than capsule preparation; try to avoid tablet preparation unless it is absolutely necessary.

Tablets can be crushed easier and usually are less expensive. I prefer the liquid, powder, or effervescent, rather than vegetarian capsules or gels, least of all tablets due to less absorption in tablets.

- **DIET**

All the above nutrition discussion would not be so important if our diet was full of the nutrition needed for our bodies. Everyone requires a different amount of calories and a different ratio of protein, fat, and sugar. In this aspect, our actual food quality is getting worse and worse. People often go for the fastest way to prepare it (such as in fast food restaurants). Many of our readily available foods are found in a package, sealed with airtight plastic and priced right for our budget.

When we are fully employed and live in a city with unpredictable traffic, we can at least prepare a good meal that we think is healthier during the weekend. Too many factors prevent us from cooking like we used to fifty years ago. Our farmers' markets now are usually only available weekly, farmers market provide locally grown products and often organic. This is preferable to products shipped from long distances. At night, after working for eight hours and two hours in traffic, which is what we have in Los Angeles where I live, we do not want to cook. I am very fortunate to have lived just fifteen minutes away from my office for more than three decades now.

Raising three children in married life and currently working full time in an office, and being responsible for many activities, I find that getting a "master chef" is a dream of any women or man who has that kind of schedule. I tried to balance this so-called diet but failed tremendously when we were busy during weekdays. During weekends, we felt like we wanted to use it to enjoy the day to catch up with what we couldn't do during weekdays. So it was difficult to eat right and prepare our own food.

Technology brings our world so close together and all work becomes more efficient and done in a faster way and timelier manner. This kind of speed makes everyone nervous if they have to cook. The best is still having one person who goes to work and the other spouse who takes care of the house, children, and the diet of course. How fortunate is a family that has had this luxury in the last ten years, or perhaps twenty years. Many families have to have both parents go to work to survive.

Our basic rule of thumb for healthy aging diet is very simple.

1. More protein (vegetable source is best, seeds, nuts, legumes, or small amount of grass-fed or organic meat. We need about 50–70 grams of protein daily depending on your size. That can be absorbed easily from vegetables, like kale, broccoli, bok choy, beans, nuts, seeds, berries and fruits, and fish, like wild-caught salmon.

   When you add a protein supplement, you can use whey but there are a lot of good vegetable proteins like pea protein or gluten free plant proteins. Soy protein is harder to be absorbed. Tofu/ Tempeh fermented ones or miso are more easily absorbed. The Asians tolerate this better for some reason. They often grow up eating tofu.

2. Eat less carbohydrate using (unrefined carbohydrate, fiber and low glycemic is best)

3. Eat less fats, eat unsaturated fat, omega 3, flaxseed, and fish

The ratio should be 50 percent protein, 25 percent carbohydrates preferable complex (vegetables), and 25 percent fat, preferably good oil like coconut, uncured meat, and unsaturated fat like avocado and olive oils.

Some people have decided to grow their own vegetables and also keep hens to get fresh eggs daily at home. This is not possible in the cities with many in condominium housing.

A ratio of 50:25:25 (Protein: Carbohydrate: fat) is good. Basically you want to go light on the following:

1. Rice (brown rice preferred). I use quinoa instead as a grain.
2. Pasta, all kinds. I use the angel hair or glass noodle or vermicelli.
3. Breads, all kinds. I try to use the one that is gluten free or full multigrain wheat instead of white.

4. Avoid desserts especially sweet ones, except low glycemic sugar ones like apple, pears, berries, and peaches.
5. Avoid sweet drinks as sugary and soda based. I would use lemon squeezed in good filtered mineral water, or a sugar free drink or tea like unprocessed coconut water or all the flower teas such as chamomile, chrysanthemum, passionfruit, green tea, or nonfermented tea).
6. Sweets cause our bodies to become acidic. An acidic body would lead us to be more prone to conditions such as infections, viral infections, bacterial, yeast, and also accelerates aging. The acid-forming foods are sugary, red meats, wheat products, coffee, vinegar, and so forth. We need more alkaline food or drink. Alkaline foods are ripe fruits, apples, pears, peaches, berries, and plums, and coconut juices. The ideal is to have a pH of 7.2. You can test your pH with strips from the drug store.
7. Avoid pasteurized milk and cheeses or dairy products unless they are organic and pure.
8. Avoid all sugars and sweeteners; use stevia leaves or agave or raw honey.
9. Avoid all cereals except All Bran. There is good granola with no sugar and is gluten free.

As we age, when we eat we have to remember that our organs need a light and regular meal and moderate amount—not too much and not too little. In fact if you can, just eat only until you are 60 percent full. This is the best way and do it slowly enough so your brain will tell you that you are actually full. It takes about twenty minutes for the brain to recognize that your bodies has enough food while you are eating.

Of course, three to four small meals a day is best. But as I already said, if you cannot do this, you should supplement the meal with good food nutraceuticals. This way, you can still eat one or two times/day with one or two food supplementations in between. This way you keep a better balance in nutrition.

If you can have a choice, of course you can ask to have:

1. Immunology testing against your IgG for delayed reaction of food and vegetable or spices (Allergy testing through blood samples).
2. Nutritional evaluation and essential elements and toxic elements evaluation from blood and urine samples.
3. Blood typing is helpful.
4. The symptoms-relevant testing such as yeast, virus, bacteria, or even function of the gastrointestinal system.

The frequency:

Eat a combination of organic, fresh vegetables if possible, meat, fish, poultry, fruits, and seed or nuts mixed with spices and organic herbs. Don't eat the same food more than twice a week. This is called a rotational diet, which gives us a chance for our digestive tract to be stimulated and less irritated by the same irritable food. This kind of diet does not come easy, but we should try our best during our grocery shopping. Eat less if the good groceries are more expensive. It is better to eat less but healthier rather than more of unhealthy meals.

This book will not show you how to cook or eat in detail, but in general you should have the idea after reading this. Healthy diets can lead us to healthy aging or prolonged healthy life. There are so many organic cook books and also those that give you the number of calories just in case you are trying to cut the calories for better diet in a diabetic condition.

Heavy metals like mercury occur in seafood. Yes, basically all fishes available in the market have more than the toxic level of mercury. Although we know the wild-caught, deep-sea fishes are better, but nowadays, we do not know where in the world people have caught these fish. Nor do we know if the boat or ship passed through oil sludge. How do they catch it then? Certainly they are not swimming or flying. Their boat has to be as they should have to go to the deep sea. But I still would encourage paying attention when buying fish. Wild caught in the deep ocean is best. Hopefully they are less contaminated with mercury and other toxins.

I might throw some good recipes and healthy ones in one of the recipe chapters. Definitely you know by now that there is only one single rule of thumb that you cannot forget in this chapter. What is the one thing you should remember about refined sugar? *Eliminate* refined sugar completely. It causes illness and worse yet, cancer cells like sugar. Sugar stimulates insulin release from the pancreas, and it causes hypoglycemia, insulin resistance, and obesity or diabetes. It can also be linked to dental disease or cavities, high blood pressure, and atherosclerosis due to the irritation or inflammatory effects. Sugar can also cause osteoporosis.

Food can help people heal and can be the best medication if eaten properly. Choose the food that can provide health—the one that makes you feel good and full of energy. Don't eat food that gives you low energy and a situation where you might have go into a "food coma." When you are insulin resistant, this situation happens, and you have no energy or power to do anything after eating.

Food that is cooked too much does not produce much energy. Chinese food usually is best eaten when it is still fresh. The fishes are still swimming when you order them. Some of them are caught in the fish tank and brought in the bucket to your very eyes to examine its freshness. They believe fresh food prepared is best. Leftover food to be eaten days after is not a healthy food.

Powering Source Foods:

Vegetarian:

- Organic soy foods: tofu/tempeh
- Grains, multigrain, brown rice, gluten-free, multigrain bread, quinoa
- Organic cruciferous vegetables
- Organic dry beans and lentils
- Organic raw almonds

Animals:

- Organic Eggs
- Flaxseed oil with cottage cheese
- Unsweetened yogurt
- Organic fresh nonpasteurized milk
- Clean fish
- Organic lean meat and poultry

According to research and studies reported by numerous scientists, calorie restriction will result in prolonged healthy aging.

In my practice I encourage quarterly fasting. Eating one meal per day and two meals using a packet of minerals & protein powder and amino acid. These replacements would contain ingredients that also detox the liver and kidney to create a better homeostasis. Not only that, the patients are healthier and cleaner in their systems from toxins, but we also train them slowly how to eat less and feel good. Our goal is to eliminate the craving for sweets and sugar.

Drs. Roth and Wolford from UCLA show through the experiments in 1970s that we create a maximum metabolic balance by restricting calories. Basically you must eat a high-density, nutrient-rich diet which comes from vegetables, raw preferred, and enough protein.

We try to do it periodically, so we do not introduce too obvious of a change in diet restriction. Two weeks calorie restriction and detoxification every three months would be a good start for everyone. During the two weeks we want to restrict as much as 30–40 percent each day. If you eventually can eat less than 60 percent for two weeks every three months, you are going to detox much better and easier. Your body starts breaking down the unnecessary fats during the phase 2 detoxification, and the liver and kidneys move toxins to the urine and fecal products.

Some nutrients deplete because of properly prescribed medication. For example:

1. Antibiotic deplete: vitamin B, calcium, magnesium, orin, probiotics, inositol, other skin minerals like boron and molybdenum
2. Steroid medication deplete such as medrol and prednisone: vitamin C, vitamin D, calcium and also vitamin B
3. Dilantin (Phenytoin): vitamins B, D, K, calcium, folic acid
4. Glucophage (Metformin): vitamin B
5. NSAID (Motrin, Nuprine, Aleve, Celebrex, Tornado): folic acid, niacin, vitamin B, enzymes, hydrochloric acid
6. Antihistamine: vitamins C, B
7. Cough syrups (alcohol): vitamins B, A, biotin, cokine, folate
8. Depakote: carnitine, folic acid

My advice is to read the side effects of the drugs that you need to take more than three to six months. For short-term use, if you need to use a properly prescribed drug, please do not hesitate as conventional medicine is not a medicine that was born yesterday, either, but it is an area where we have to use with caution. We still have to know that they have their special place in our health management. They are at their best when it comes to an emergency. People cannot detoxify well when they are unable to urinate or defecate.

The conventional doctors are the best professionals at the emergency room, and all their trained staff are very skillful. Without them, you won't be safe at any time if our organs are exposed to an external insult and when natural healing does not take place. One has to be smart enough to think whether it is an emergency, urgent care, or you can read this book first and hopefully avoid having to rush to the hospital in an emergency.

****

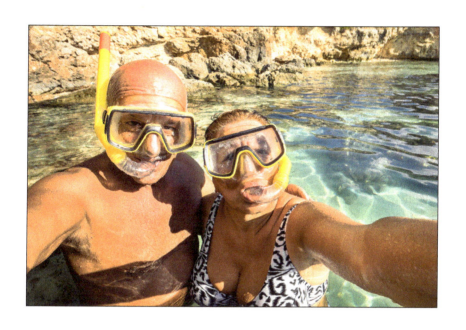

You cannot discover new oceans, unless you have the courage to lose the sight of the shore.

-Linda Jones -
Chicken soup for mother's Soul 2

Pillar III
EXERCISE and ACTIVITY

As I grow older, I actually do far less exercise than when I was in my teens or mid-twenties. I thought it was just me because I went to medical school (not an excuse actually), and in my case I moved to a different country, so all my routine has changed. Then I got married—worse, as I entered a residency program and had children (not an excuse, either, but where do I find the time?). Then I started my own practice, and my children started school, so we needed to take them to the school although it was close by. So all of these are excuses I can use, and I am sure millions of other people do the same.

Is it that important to exercise? Yes, the answer is a big yes because studies has shown that exercising regularly can improve cardiovascular functions, structure and lower blood fats such as cholesterol, strengthen bones, and regulates blood sugar much better than taking any medication or supplements. Also studies have proven that exercising regularly can improve your quality of life by improving one's organs and reduction of stress hormones. In the past twenty years, many health clubs or gyms and fitness centers are popping up everywhere. People are more aware that exercise can improve their health and prolong life.

You must continue to exercise even if you have started when you were young because in numerous studies, people become less and less able to exercise due to increasing responsibility at work, home, and with family. By the age of forty (entering the clinical stage of aging), the people who do not exercise on a regular basis would then find their health is less optimal. This is the best tool or pillar, but it is not easy.

Some people love to exercise. But for many others, it is stressful to exercise. There are different kinds of characteristics in people, which actually develop during our teens due to their parent's influences. If you train your children from the time they are young to exercise, they will like it but if not, it is more difficult to do exercise because it requires a discipline and a certain kind of sophistication to understand the right exercise.

It is not difficult in the sense that you have to know a science but a wrong exercise can also create a problem. Such as heavy weight exercises can damage some structures of ligaments or muscles. Simple instruction on the machines or proper training can help people establish a safe routine, and you can develop your understanding. Good results will follow. Once a person decides to do a routine of exercises and continues into their old age, they can easily restore their health and prolong healthy aging. Studies show people even in their eighties and nineties benefit greatly from regular exercise especially resistance or weight training.

Positive Effects of Exercise:

1. It can inhibit prevent the catabolic effects of tearing down in aging. This includes the liver and kidney function for detoxification.
2. Improves appetite, helps metabolism, and increase the high-density lipids (HDL) that can protect us from cardiovascular accidents.
3. Improves aerobic capacity and lung volume and the tone of the muscles.
4. Slows down the loss of aerobic capacity on older aging persons.
5. Both men and women benefit with the same effects.
6. Improves bone density for sure and helps strengthens the bones.
7. Improves body composition.

Too much exercise can harm our tissues. There can be negative effects to our healthy aging situation if you force your exercise beyond the regular "healthy exercise zone" because it produces stress to the body. This stress can cause the increase of cortisol, which accelerates aging. Intense exercise regularly actually reduces our immune system because it reduces our natural killer cells from the T lymphocytes or the white blood cells. Marathon or ultra-long distance races are examples of too much exercise at once.

The Goals of Exercise for Healthy Aging

1. Improve your balance
2. Become more flexible
3. Maintain or improve the strength in your muscles.

Types of Healthy Aging Exercises That We Can Combine

1. Flexibility. Set aside one third of your exercise time for range of motion and flexibility training. As we age, our flexibility and balance is reduced, as well as muscle bulk. If we don't keep ourselves limber and flexible, we might fall.

2. Strengthening exercise is to maintain our muscle tone. This kind of exercise is called weight-training exercise. This also improves bone density. This type of exercise also stimulates the production of human growth hormone, which is also considered a Fountain of Youth hormone. This is the part that prolongs healthy aging.

3. Cardiovascular exercises maintain the "ejection fraction" percentage, which is the amount of blood that squeezes out of the heart to circulate in our bodies and brain. This will prolong healthy aging, as the oxygen will make our cells breathe better. This can be walking, jogging, air bicycling, or regular stationary if not outdoor bicycle, etc.

4. Cognitive, or brain, exercise is to stimulate our memories to stay sharp and quick in recalling memories. Our brain is very complex in function, and it does require exercise, since it is one of our important organs that need maintenance.

This exercise includes reading a good book with some stories or what is happening in the news, doing word puzzles, and playing games with multiplication of space configurations. Playing board games (can be longer than electronic games as it does not emit EMF–electro magnetic fields), or sport games that requires technique such as Ping-Pong and sport board. Exercise with Chess, Mah Jong, or Bridge can be very helpful. There are many other fun routines you can actually develop such as following programs like *Would You Like to Be a Millionaire* and *Family Feud* on television. Involving yourself in answering those questions stimulates your brain function.

It is so important to maintain brain function because there is no point of living longer if you can't remember things (Alzheimer's or memory impairment). Like who was that pretty gal who kissed me?

5. Colon (Digestive tract) exercising. This is part of our bodies that is called a "second brain." Basically it is the part of our digestive system, and it extends from the cecum (where your appendix is and where the gastrocolonic reflex ends) to ascending, transverse, and descending colon, passing the sigmoid before the rectum and finally exiting the anus "door."

From the cecum to the anus, this area is where our final waste products rest, waiting for the healthy gastrocolonic reflex to move them out or the "gravity effect." At night detoxification happens in the liver and kidneys. If you do not eat late at night, your bodies can have a chance to detoxify your colon.

Healthy bowel movement is when you can move your content (waste products) within two hours of your input or meal. Therefore, if you eat once a day, you move once but for three meals, you should see three movements.

The movement is important, but the most important is the volume. Although we do not discuss this here in detail, I want to touch this area in this book because it is so important that you might not have a good brain if this area is not clean.

After you eat, you should be able to have the urge to go within two hours. This urge should not be suppressed, and you should normally look for a nearby rest room so you can relax having your bowel movement and the cleansing of your colon. Should you plan to suppress this urge, then you are training your brain function and body to go against your natural gastrocolonic reflex.

This reflex can be put off but only for so long. Most people lose this and will not have that normal urge after meals when they grow up. Only a small percentage of healthy people will find a routine bowel movement during their adult age. Not too many doctors will ask about your bowel habits. It was part of my problem, which I discovered during my unhealthy years of my late teens. So I appreciate the solution, and I am giving it back to my patients as part of my initial evaluation.

Colon cleansing is one of the best detoxes I have ever experienced in my practice and life. I experienced all kinds of colon cleansing before I finally concluded after many years that the open hydrocolonic is lifesaving. Why do I say that? It is because 80 percent of our defense mechanism of our immune system is focused on keeping the toxic material out of our colon, and to prevent spill back into our bodies system through the mechanism called the mesentericum.

This mesh is complicated and sophisticated; architecturally it looks like a spider web but has the best and the most important job in our bodies. They are our police.

Together with the friendly bacteria, they both keep us alive and healthy.

Diet and nutrition can be used to influence this function for sure. No matter how much you move if you have a period of life where you only move a smaller amount of waste products compared to the amount of food you eat, then the rest is stuck in your colon wall and everywhere else. What will you do if waste is stuck there? Well you can suffocate the wall area and cause an impairment of function in absorption and synthesis with some chemical like sterol. It is very important that we check this function in our routine to determine if your gastrointestinal system is healthy.

Science has discovered that the initial source of trouble to our health usually starts in the gastrointestinal tract. I think everyone agrees, as we have to eat on a regular basis to generate our fuel and be able to function normally. I don't think we can argue that one of the reasons that we start our clinical aging stage at age forty years is because we can't detox well. This is what I am talking about. If you keep the real toxins in your bodies for years, it is only natural that we need a few months or years to reverse the situation.

Using drugs for constipation is a mistake in my opinion. If you want to medicate this area with natural products before it gets too late then we need to look into something like colon cleansing (hydrocolonic—the open system for healthy aging). We offer this services and many patients have enjoyed good outcomes from it. The closed system can be used for elderly who can't even walk or also debilitated patients.

Basically if you do an open system, you need someone who can understand simple instruction and also wants to do this for health. We include other aids if need be such as fibers, enzymes, probiotics, and good amounts of water.

6   Skin exercise for the aesthetic appearance is commonly done. More people start early with healthy skin hygiene. It is important not to put too many chemical products on your skin to keep it healthy. Many natural skin preparations are available in the market.

Most important like many organs, exercise here is giving some tension and pressure to our skin. For the face, a facial is one of them, acupressure, detoxification can be the exercise.

Prolonging healthy aging definitely is easier if you know how to keep this pillar moving. This is the only pillar that is very affordable or can be done without supervision by doctors or therapists.

****

PILLAR IV
STRESS REDUCTION

Stress can kill and is powerful. Although it is commonly understood, it can be misunderstood. People always think stress has to be unhappy. Stress does not mean you have to be unhappy. Stress is part of a normal life. Stress has a close link to chemicals in our bodies like cortisol, adrenalin, GABA, epinephrine, or norepinephrine, serotonin, and genetic involvement.

This is why you want to read this kind of book because you need to know how to help your primary care doctor to see if you have this kind of condition. It is going to be a waste of time unless you have a good primary care physician who can help you maintain your healthy aging. Long life is not the standard you want to achieve. Healthy long life is what our goal is if you want to live a long productive life.

There Are Four Kinds of Simple Categories of STRESS.

1. **"Happy Stress"**

    This kind of stress is the most dangerous stress because you don't know that your stress is going to affect your health negatively.

    Examples of this type of stress:

- Athletes who train vigorously to meet their next goal of success in their field and compete for a prize and achievement.
- Researchers who are meeting their due date to qualify for their next grant. Working under tight schedule but love what they do in their work.
- Musicians who handle their instruments in a stretched negative ergonomic posture.
- Dancers who abuse their joints through their movement in those fast movements.

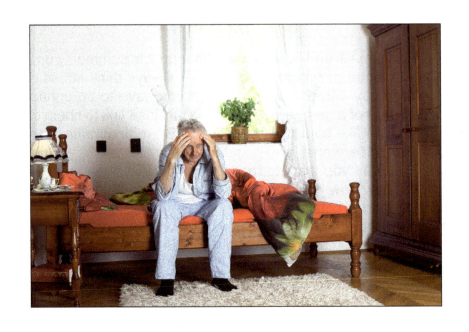

*So whatever is wrong
With your life today,
You'll find a solution
If you kneel down and pray.
Not just for pleasure,
Enjoyment, and health,
Not just for honors and prestige and wealth.
But pray for a purpose to make life worth living.*

—H. S. Rice

- Pilots with odd hours who have to always fly across the meridian lines and adapt constantly to the changing of times.
- Those artists or campers who work under a certain heat and nonsupportive environment such as "burning man" campers in Nevada
- Archeologists who understand that they are going to a toxic environment area to find their "treasure."
- The martial arts people, or body builders who train their body and muscular skeletal organs to go to the next level and beyond normal achievement.
- Missionaries who try to satisfy their spiritual goal and go too far to claim their success.
- Ring sports like boxing.
- Mountain climbers
- Bungee jumpers
- Sky divers
- Scuba divers
- Don't forget writers, editors, and proofreaders who are under the gun, as well.

You can understand now what I mean by happy stress. These people are happily doing what they do but stressing their health and creating unhealthy conditions. Most of them realize this before they go into this field, but they "love it," they "want" it, "they like it," and they are "happy" to see that result, even knowing it might hurt their health. These categories can be called "stress with awareness." These groups of people should read this book so they can prevent or minimize damage when it comes.

They should:

1. Take enough extra supplements for the organs they overuse.
2. Should change their schedule to retire three to five years earlier to establish their own aging markers. They age faster than normal people
3. Detoxify routinely.

4. Never miss their annual comprehensive healthy aging screening.

2. Mental Stress

This type of stress can be self-inflicted, genetic factors, or an unavoidable part of life. Both physical and psychological damage can be the result. In this category, you can name any type of stress, and it will fit because this is the common kind of stress that people understand.

Problems, yes problems, are usually what they think the cause is. It can be with their coworkers, loved ones, boyfriends, girlfriends, parents or siblings, government, politics, war, bad or good news, or just as simple as bad traffic on the way to their daily work. Tight schedules, children in home, work involvement, bad weather, problems in the neighborhood, and so forth can all cause stress. Many people can handle it well and lessen the effect of the stress, but many create even more complicated situations when they are under stress.

The result of this stress can change the body composition and chemicals

1. Being irritable, fatigued and be unable to sleep with no energy and loss of libido due to hormone changes.
2. Memory loss due to lack of vitamins B, C, and other supportive minerals.
3. Headache due to lack of sleep and loss of minerals.
4. Breathing problems due to prolonged poor posture.
5. High blood pressure.
6. Gastrointestinal changes, like diarrhea, bloating, constipation, and gas.

All of those symptoms quickly can affect the healthy aging states.

3. Pharmaceutical Stress

This is people who are put on long-term drugs or people who are using drugs as recreational reasons. Not too smart! These people are abusing their brain and pituitary glands. When it inhibits the production of HGH (Human Growth Hormone) then the HGF (Human Growth Factors) are depleted. This is the stage where your DNA telomerase can become shortened and your life span is shortened

4. Environmental Stress

Since I use the whole house water filtration system to get our source of clean water for daily use, I feel that our health has improved. This is the price we pay to live in a metropolitan city where our air, water, and food are contaminated compared to moving to Tianmen Mountain in China or Hunza.

This stress affects healthy aging in many ways. All our cells react to stress because stress releases chemicals as cortisol and adrenaline. Under stress our pituitary gland produces more of our ACTH (adrenocorticotropic hormone). This is a precursor to the cortisol cortisone. These are two stress hormones, which inhibit the immune system from working well. All kinds of stress responds the same in physiological responses.

When the stress hormones go up, the response is to metabolize protein, fat, and carbohydrates faster. This is the process that produces energy. When your organs work extra miles to produce this cortisol or stress hormone, that is an extra load and your organs can become exhausted. While stress is part of your daily life, you must ask yourself how you are going to cope with this to avoid the damage to your health.

I am going to give you some tips that have evidence-based science behind them so you can protect against the exhaustion of your chemical system in your bodies.

The focus is the *goal*. Remember the goal is to *reduce* it, not to *erase it*. It is impossible, I think, to erase all stress in our lives. The goal is to recognize it and to be in charge of it, which means that you have to find a solution to help the reduction of your stress. One of them is, of course, to find the doctor who is willing to work with you. In my practice, I test their blood first when they come regardless of who it is because people's tolerance of stress is different. This can be measured.

Once I measure the blood work if it is not the right number, even if they feel good and healthy, it is not wise to keep quiet and not do anything. You might run on "reserve," and one day when that reserve is gone, you will collapse. This reserve system is just like the sign on your car dashboard measuring the level of gas in the gas tank of the car you drive. When the light is yellow telling you that your gasoline is low in the tank, the reserve sign starts to show that you are using the reserve gasoline. Certain cars can run further than other cars. In my car I think I have about twenty miles before the car stops.

It is similar to our bodies. While your numbers are showing too high in your blood test, you might not feel any problem. However, your experienced doctor will tell you and suggest something that you should start paying attention to in order to save your healthy aging life. I hope this is clear enough as this pillar can kill faster than other pillars. In fact, it is this pillar that can work like firecrackers and spread everywhere out of control. Due to the external factors, this pillar is the only pillar that you can't fix yourself. I would say, this can be the most expensive pillar if you don't handle it soon enough.

Now you know that all humans need certain stress to move up and grow. Without this stress, people would not have any motivation, and this would probably be a boring world. Most productive people who can survive stress are those who are more successful. The daily stress management in life and the maintaining of the body reactions is the key to the pillar of reduction of stress. There are many ways to easily reduce the big factors that seem small.

Those are:

- Mental activities to reduce psychological stress such as listening to music, reading books, playing instruments, or watching nice movies have a calming effect.
- Functional activities can reduce stress for people who love going to spas, having a massage for myofascial release to help our circulation.
- Those who use physical activities to reduce stress can enjoy gardening, shopping, fishing, driving, and walking; simple breathing exercises help.
- Deep breathing is part of the technique used in the ancient Chinese exercises called Tai Chi and Qi Gung. They exercise an energy source using a breathing technique. Try breathing in for 4 seconds fill your chest in full then hold it for 4 seconds. Then release the air slowly for 6 seconds and don't breath 2 seconds and repeat 10 times da day.

  In western dancing and singing, deep breathing is a must. And also in much competitive exercise, breathing technique is basic for their exercise.

Many other techniques cannot be proven by science, but they work. More studies will confirm and bring them to scientific clinical evidence.

1. Spiritual healing (for those who believe) will use this as a first resort because they believe that their God is the greatest Healer.

   Many people, who don't believe in or don't have time for God, still use meditation techniques. They do not have any religious factors, but this meditation calms them.

2. Medical hypnotherapy (for people who smoke, alcoholics and drug addicts).

3. Earthling therapy (should soon be proven scientifically) is using the Earth's gravity to normalize our homeostasis of the healthy aging stage. A good book on this is called *Earthling* by Dr. Stephen Sinatra MD (he is an Integrative Cardiologist).

4. Urine and Fecal Transplant (based on excess bio-nutrition) that helps people who can only receive nutrition from biological products.

Any techniques or special treatments, if you do not embrace them on a long-term basis, will not work in the long term. Daily practice makes this pillar become the most effective pillar after all. You did not get ill quickly, and it will take time to recover your health.

When you are stressed, your metabolism can slow down, and many get tense and even forget to drink enough water or to eat enough. Therefore you know if you skip meals, you need to drink more water. Supplementation of nutraceuticals would be meaningful if you skip meals to improve healthy aging.

Environment at Home Can also Help

1. Maintain the home so that you enjoy going there after work or during weekends.
2. Keep the noise level as low as possible or have nice music throughout the day.
3. Natural lighting or yellow light is better than white fluorescent light for relaxation.
4. In your home environment, you must try to reduce your anxiety levels to a minimum on a daily basis.
5. Fix the electromagnetic and "dirty electricity" energy that can cause interruption of the central nervous system and also the immune system. *Dirty Electricity* is a book by Samuel Milham that can help you understand the dangers. Certain devices can be use to reduce this problems

Sleep Hygiene during Rest Periods

- Take early dinner so your stomach activities are as low as possible at night.
- Empty your bladder before bedtime.
- Stop water intake after 7:00 PM
- Take all medication before dinner.
- Turn off all lights and have no blue light at all (TV button light, cell phone, laptop).
- Try not to watch TV in your bedroom.
- Do not stay in bed if you can't sleep within twenty to thirty minutes. Get up and read my book or the Bible. Try Deuteronomy—that will put you out.
- Try to use sleep aids such as melatonin-slow release, phenibut, valerian root, magnesium (to relax the muscles), sedalia, chamomile, serotonin, kava kava, and so forth.

****

Needless Worry

Some of your hurts you have cured,
And the sharpest you still have survived
But what torments of grief you endured
From evils which never arrived !

-Ralph Waldo Emerson-

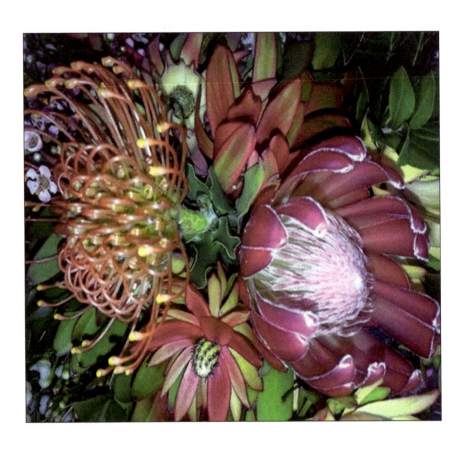

And if today is cloudy,
Tomorrow might be fine.
No one has ever failed who kept
A happy state of mind.

The longest journey taken
Starts with a single smile,
And one-day-at-a-time can change
The worthless to hormone balancing—that is worthwhile!

—Salesian Mission

Pillar V
HORMONE BALANCING

The endocrine (hormone) system is the what, who, how, which, when and where system. In this chapter you will find a basic concept of what a hormone is, how you can balance your hormones, why do you need hormone supplements, which hormone is good for you, who is going to help you with these sensitive issues, and where you can find them?

Let's start with **what?**

Hormones are a substance produced by our bodies in very small amounts. They are chemicals, and they are small. They are very potent chemicals and can have a high impact on our health.

How?

Hormones work in our bodies as biochemical messengers, facilitating communication between every cell in our bodies. They are essential to making our lives lively, beautiful, strong, and sexual. Their production is influenced by other chemicals, such as enzymes, minerals, vitamins, proteins, and genetic status.

How do we balance them?

Certainly there are many hormones that work synergistically or inhibit the others when they function. The organs that produce hormones are called glandular organs.

Where?

Here is the list and where they are produced:

Pituitary glands

- Luteinizing hormone (LH)

- Follicle stimulating hormone (FSH)
- Growth hormone (GH)
- Adrenocorticotrophic hormone (ACTH)
- Lipothropin, endorphin
- Thyroid-stimulating hormone (TSH)
- Melanocyte-stimulating hormone
- B-endorphin
- Vasopressin
- Diuretic hormone
- Oxytocin

Thyroid

- Thyroxin
- Trioiodothyronine
- Calcitonin

Parathyroid

- Parathyroid Hormone

Thymus

- Thyroxin factors, Thymic factors, Thymulin
- Thymopetin

Adrenal

- Cortisol, aldosterone
- DHEA (Dehydropiandrosterone)
- Androstenedione
- Epinephrine
- Norepinephrine

Gonads

- Testosterone

- Estradiol
- Androstenedione
- Inhibit
- Activin
- Mullerian inhibiting substance

OVARIES:

- Progesterone
- Estrogen (Estrone, Estradiol, Estriol)
- Androstenedione
- Inhibin and activin
- Follicle releasing (FS) peptide
- Relaxin

Placenta

- Human chorionic gonadotropin hormone (HCGH)
- Human placenta lactogen (HPL)
- Progesterone
- Estrogen

PANCREAS

- Insulin
- Glucagon
- Somatostatin
- Pancreatic polypeptide
- Gastrin
- Vasoactive intestinal peptide (VIP)

PINEAL

- Melatonin
- Biogenic amines
- Peptides

We don't usually check all these hormones at once, but in my practice I check the hormone of each glandular function. When the patient comes in with symptoms, I check in detail to find out if their organs are experiencing a serious condition that triggers the symptoms. Since hormones have such an important function in facilitating the cellular communications, it is a physician's job to make sure that this is part of their checklist when they see their patients.

Unfortunately there is not a specialist called "Hormone Specialist." A physician or medical doctor practicing medicine should know how to handle this area. To a certain degree, the endocrinologist is probably the specialist you need to see for metabolic diseases. They might not try to balance your sex hormones as they might think it is the duty of an organ specialist.

Unfortunately, brain surgeons/neurosurgeons and neurologists are the physicians who do not deal with any hormone imbalances.

The OBGYN physicians usually are the most expected to deal with hormones, since they deal with the placenta, the uterus, and the ovaries. They only want to make sure that your uterus and your ovaries are healthy. They rarely check hormones at your annual follow-up visit. They want to check to see if you have any gynecological problems. If your vaginal mucosa is dry, then they will give you estradiol. They are the ones who first announce that you have a cancer of your cervix or uterus.

Hormone activity begins with the fetal stage in the womb and extends through our entire life.

Hormone Insufficiency Symptoms Are:

1. Loss of muscle tone
2. Loss of strength
3. Fatigue
4. Depression
5. Memory loss
6. Osteopenia or osteoporosis
7. Reduced skin elasticity
8. Gray hair

9. Reduced sexual libido
10. Dryness of mucous membranes and genital area
11. Frequent yeast infections or UTI
12. Uncontrolled weight gain
13. Irritability
14. Mood swings
15. Wrinkles
16. Thinning hair
17. Constipation
18. Brittle nails
19. Insomnia
20. Cardiovascular symptoms
21. Hypertension
22. Weak immune system

PEAK PRODUCTION

Most of our hormones peak at the age of twenty. For women, hormones peak at the age of seventeen to nineteen. Boy's hormones peak at the age of twenty to twenty-five. This is proportionate to the production of the growth hormone, and it peaks at that point, then starts to decline after that age.

HUMAN GROWTH HORMONE

The famous healthy-aging hormone is called the Fountain of Youth or the Human Growth Hormone. Another name for this is the *master hormone* or the anti-aging hormone. We do not know how it works after growth has maximized itself at a certain age. Girls maximize growth at the age of seventeen to nineteen and boys at age twenty to twenty-five. After the peak, the hormone release is decreased by 14 percent every ten years until age sixty or seventy when advanced aging leaves us with just 10–15 percent of the healthy level that we might want to maintain.

HGH–Human Growth Hormone—is a peptide hormone that has 191 amino acids in a single polypeptide chain. It is produced by the pituitary gland in the brain, and it is a response to hypothalamus stimulation called growth hormone releasing hormone (GHRH). All other hormones are also a complex secretion of these two glands.

The end product of HGH is the IGF-1 Insulin Growth Factor-1 (Somatomedin–C) that is released through the liver. This is measured in the serum and also bound to a different protein called IgF-BP3. Also it is measured and monitored for HGH supplementation treatment.

Daniel Rudman, who studied and reported his findings in the NEJM (New England Journal of Medicine) in 1968, marked the development of the era of anti-aging medicine. This led to hormone replacement for healthy aging.

They understand now we do not need a double-blind study, just like many other conventional medicine procedures, for example, by-pass surgery in the cardiac surgery field. We have no double-blind studies, yet our results can be scientifically documented through testing and measured objective findings. Hormone enhancements give us hope of extending life of healthy aging in general, which is the main goal, not just extending life. The declining of HGH cannot be prevented as we age. All the symptoms mark the stage of aging.

For years no one reported the real symptoms of HGH deficiency except those that measured during the retardation of a child's growth. These are necessary for the treatment of dwarfism.

For adult use, the Growth Hormone supplementation shows an improvement in:

1. Muscle strength and size
2. Loss of body fat
3. Exercise tolerance and endurance
4. Skin texture, thickness, elasticity, disappearance of wrinkles
5. Common illnesses
6. Duration of penile erection and sexual potency
7. Frequency in night time urination
8. Hot flashes
9. Energy level
10. Memory and Cognitive function

11. Muscular skeletal flexibility
12. Hair growth
13. Old injury healing

These results invite a huge interest in the medical community and among physicians themselves, but the cost is relatively expensive right now. Each unit can run about $20 to $25, and it is a daily injection.

Under my observation, the supplementation for thirty days with 1 to 2 units can sustain its benefit with a three-month break in between. Therefore the real usage is only three months in a year. Among the people who can afford this in my thirty years of practice, I only see benefits with no side effects.

SECRETAGOGUES

This is a nutraceutical product that can be used as HGH stimulators. Some people call this HGH releaser. Basically, it has a special delivery system that can absorb through a mucosal membrane, and it absorbs in seconds to stimulate the pituitary gland while we are asleep between 11:00 PM and 3:00 AM.

This secretagogues are best used when you are having a low reading on the IgF-1 (Insulin Growth factor 1) scale. If you have symptoms of insufficiency of HGH, and you have failed to improve your symptoms, after using all the precursors, and supplementing with the other hormones, then secretagogous can stimulate your anterior pituitary glandular to produce more of the biological growth hormone.

HGH use does not need secretagogues but in the period where you felt better yet cannot afford to continue taking the HGH all year round, you should take it a few months then restart it again. Based on my observation, the IgF-1 level would rise with HGH and stay at a good level controlling your symptoms for about three or four months. Then without HGH, it starts declining again. For an unknown reason, we know that aging has caused this decline, and the pituitary gland is not able to produce it as much as before. When you supplement it with real HGH injection, it increases and gives you the benefit of HGH. But due to the organ's actual capacity of producing HGH, it falls slowly again to the level where it was. It was during the time when you did not take HGH, the secretagogues helped maintain it for many long months.

You need to take secretagogues at the right time, which is in the evening before 11:00 p.m., and you have to have an empty stomach for two hours, as it is a peptide, so it competes with other proteins or sugar in your diet.

HGH can be introduced at any time. Among all the hormones, only HGH is found to have no "negative feedback" to glandular production, meaning if you take additional HGH, it is not going to make your gland be lazy and stop or inhibit production of its own glandular secretion. I personally am enjoying both of these products and have seen the benefit on my health and my complexion. I notice when I don't take the HGH for any reason. My father who is now eighty-eight years old would notice it right away, and he likes to take it daily.

The myth is that it causes cancer, and none of my patients who have been taking HGH for the past thirty years have developed any kind of cancer. My father's prostate, enlarged thirty years ago, now is a normal size, and his PSA is as normal as it can be like a young person's PSA. I am not worried about cancer. If it causes cancer then we should not give it to dwarfed children, as it would not be ethical. The pediatrician gives a high dose of HGH, as high as thirty units daily to dwarfed children to stimulate their growth for years until they see no further improvement, when they stop. Conventional medicine never had any problems with this practice, but it is when we try to help an elderly person who is helpless and has classical symptoms of low HGH that there is no approval.

You probably have to have a condition like Parkinson's syndrome, or multiple sclerosis with lethargic situation and reach about eighty years of age before insurance companies will approve partial coverage from insurance companies for the standard HGH test. Even with partial coverage, many patients, due to their age and financial situation, can't afford this excellent hormone that has a nickname of "The Master Hormone." The good news is that HGH pricing has gone down almost 50 percent from thirty years ago.

You don't have to be a Hollywood star or millionaire to afford this. You just need a physician who knows how to monitor this and give it to you with the secretagogues.

How can we name this hormone "The Master Hormone" when it is true that it can master other hormones to regulate the homeostasis and the biological needs of the system and restore energy of the person who needs it?

Let's emphasize here the Precursors DHEA-S04 and LH, FSH, and all the sexual hormones. Below is the pathway of the precursor and synthesis of steroid hormones. If we called DHEA as a mother of hormones, I would like to introduce the grandmother of hormones, which is our famous

CHOLESTEROL

Cholesterol is our source of sex hormones in the pathway and we need to have a good amount. As we age cholesterol becomes an issue because of its particles which can create plaque and cardiovascular insults. However management of cholesterol using anticholesterol "life-saving" drugs like statins should be evaluated carefully. To balance cholesterol or lipoprotein B/A ratio, we can use nutraceutical products, exercise, and select our diets properly. The side effect of statin drugs to these steroid pathways is reduction of the sexual hormone. This can cause loss of energy, mood swings, or erectile dysfunction in men. If you are not aware of this, you may review the healthy-aging pillar and restore production of sex hormones instead of taking statin drugs.

Cholesterol comes from our own body synthesis and an external source, which is diet. Once you know how to manage synthesis without taking drugs and manage your diet or triglycerides, then the big portion of the symptomatic imbalanced hormone is pretty much solved with healthy pillars.

The precursor of our sexual hormones is:

1. **DHEA (Dehydroepiandrosterone),** which is the mother of hormones.

This is the androgenic hormone that gives you energy because it is also the source of testosterone. Naturally, this is abundantly produced in our bodies, and that is why it is called the mother of hormones or mother of all sex steroids. This is the precursor of testosterone in men, and also produces more than 60–70 percent of estrogen in our premenopausal or menopausal periods.

After the menopause period, this produces almost 100 percent of estrogen in our bodies. Thus if your DHEA sources are low, your estrogen is almost zero as well as the level found in testing after menopause, and you develop all kinds of low estrogen symptoms.

Average men ages twenty-five to forty have more DHEA than women of the same age group. But after age forty or fifty, DHEA produces more estrogen than testosterone in men. In general men produce more DHEA than women even after age fifty. Maintaining DHEA levels can combat fatigue in the aging process because this precursor is also responsible for communication of many organs such as our brains and breasts, ovaries, prostate, muscles, liver, and cardiovascular cells. Some studies shows that DHEA can prevent over expression of cells sensitive to sex hormones; thus this can also be used as an anticancer medication during aging as a preventative measure.

The active metabolites are the ones I usually measure in the serum level. It is called DHEA–Sulfate. The half-life of DHEA–S04 seems to be longer than DHEA. It can easily be measured by laboratories. This is synthesized in the Adrenal cortex's ZONA reticular, where it also produces other precursors and a small amount of sex hormone. In men, 10–25 percent of the DHEA is produced by the testicles. Both men and women get some of the DHEA from their brain. Daily secretion of DHEA in our bodies is about 4 mg or 25 mg of the DHEA Sulfate.

2. **PREGNENOLONE**

Pregnenolone is the other precursor of hormones together with DHEA; this gives you more of your memory ability than energy ability. Most people never get tested on this one precursor. It is mistaken for progesterone, and some patients who are men might misunderstand this to be a woman's hormone and be confused about this excellent precursor. These precursors are directly synthesized from cholesterol in the mitochondria.

Pregnenolone is also produced in the adrenal gland as I had mentioned earlier and the brain. This is called the neuron steroid because it improves your memory in cognitive performance.

Function of Pregnenolone:

1. Positive effect on the central nervous system
2. Involved in creating neuron brain cells.
3. Helps to improve appearance
4. Improves emotional attitude
5. Precursor of sex hormones
6. Helps in restoring the neuroendocrine system.

Lack of Pregnenolone Symptoms:

- Fatigue
- Depressed mood
- Sleep problems
- Skin color is not glowing
- Stiffness or joint pains for no reason
- Declining memories

CORTISOL

Cortisol is another hormone made in the adrenals but in a different area called the Zona fasciculate. Like many of the rest of our hormones, the functions of the organs in the aging process decline accordingly and proportionate to the decline in all hormone levels. Some other factors like elevated insulin levels, enzymes, and stress in life also affect the production DHEA.

Some other *good effects of DHEA* found by scientists are:

1. Inhibits the inflammation factors such as Interleukin 6 (IL-6)
2. It is an antioxidant
3. It inhibits cytokines (pro-inflammatory factors that rise with age or with chronic inflammation)
4. It may lower blood sugar
5. It reduces the negative side effects of cortisol which rise in high-stress situations
6. It can be used as biomarker of aging in anti-aging medicine practice.

Low DHEA symptoms:

1. Lack of hair such as pubic hair and underarm hair or eye brows
2. Depressed mood with anxiety
3. Weak muscle and lack of muscle tone
4. Usually can't tolerate noises
5. Lack of sexual libido
6. Dry skin, dry eyes, and dry and brittle hair
7. Poor memory

Many scientists believe that the cause of some of the chronic diseases is adrenal exhaustion. Because they always found a low DHEA–S level in those with chronic immune system issues or cancer and autoimmune patients. Low DHEA is when you have this condition but it is not the cause of these conditions. The use of cortisol to suppress arthritic conditions of other autoimmune conditions can lower DHEA levels

MELATONIN

Produced by the pineal gland, bone marrow, and intestinal tract. It is referred to as the *biological clock* because it buffers or paces our hormones. It is called the light-and-dark situation. The night and day is called Circadian Rhythm or often also is referred the as biorhythms of the body.

Function of Melatonin in Our System for Healthy Aging

1. Biological need such as sexual activity and fertility
2. Antioxidant effects
3. Protects DNA from oxidative damage
4. Inhibits viral replication
5. Protects the body from infection
6. Anticancer properties
7. Sleep and awake regulators
8. Hunger and thirst regulators
9. As a neuroprotectant and anti-inflammatory both, it might have great treatment effect on Alzheimer's disease.
10. Part of the role of healthy aging, it deters the aging process

It is closely related to the neurochemical called serotonin (in the brain as well). Tryptophan (5 HTP Hydroxytryptophan) is an amino acid, which is the precursor of serotonin which then becomes the precursor of melatonin.

Melatonin is suppressed by light and increased by darkness. That is why it is very important to make sure that it is "jet black" dark when you sleep so you get abundant melatonin. Scientists also believe visual stimulation before you go to sleep such as watching television or with the bright light on is the cause of depletion of melatonin. Its production peaks between 1:00 to 4:00 AM. If you are not asleep in the dark by then, the production is poor.

Melatonin is also a good hormone that will inhibit the growth of cancer cells and promote apoptosis or the program of cell death (commit suicide) in the cancer cell system. In Russia, Melatonin in a high dose, like 40–50 mg, is used to treat cancer.

Low melatonin symptoms:

1. Difficulty sleeping
2. Abnormal sleep pattern like having jet lag
3. Having difficulty falling back to sleep after waking up in the middle of the night.
4. Feeling out of it, lack of feeling well.

5. Having a problem tolerating thyroid symptoms, low free T3
6. Body temperature either too hot or too cold at night
7. Premature grey hair
8. Having difficulty waking up in the morning

THYROID

Thyroid has a nick name called the "great imitator." Thyroid is produced by the thyroid gland that is located in the neck area and it is usually palpable when you hold your front neck area by the air pipe. It is as big as an apricot seed. Why it is called the great imitator? When the thyroid hormone is low, the person will have all kinds of symptoms that mimic other conditions.

If it is just slightly low, because of its ability to control almost every chemical reaction in our bodies, it can cause:

1. Impaired metabolism
2. Impaired immune system
3. Low energy
4. Weight gain due to increase in fat
5. Foggy brain
6. Getting sick easily
7. Yeast infection and bacterial infection
8. Increased risk of cancer.
9. Symptoms of aging diseases

Many scientists and physicians have agreed that hypothyroidism can be subclinical, meaning, you may not see a low level in your lab results, but you can have symptoms already. My opinion is the standard value in the lab result has not been changed for decades, and the range is so narrow that patients who really have a problem can be very sick already before the number of free T3 falls below the lowest range.

The biggest problem is also that conventional prescriptions are usually a T4 base (Thyroxin), and if your bodies works well, the T4 is converted by your bodies to produce T3 and then methylated to free T3, which you can use. Since there was no T3 material in the past and most of the prescriptions used during our conventional training was T4, you don't actually get to experience using T3 (triiodothyronine), which is widely available now if you are an endocrinologist physician.

The most frustrating part is that the testing for Free T3 has not been part of the panel you order in the laboratories. You need to request this separately unless the laboratories support the integrative practice. Many of my patients who were referred by their friends, came with a report from their physician and it only has TSH. The practice in the old days was when your Thyroid hormone was low usually it made the TSH (thyroid-stimulating hormone to work harder and it would show a higher level. The problem is that checking only TSH does not mean showing a patient has enough free T3, which is the hormone that you need to be picked up by the receptor cells to be used by the cell. Free T3 is also a biomarker of the aging condition.

Why care if the TSH is normal? Probably the patient has a problem that does not elevate the TSH until they have clinical full-blown hypothyroidism. Thyroid care is complex, and we have to be careful not to aggravate a condition where the patient can also develop Hashimoto's where the thyroid hormone is too high, becomes excessive for a long period of time, and it attacks their own immune system.

Another common condition is Grave's disease (Thyrotoxicosis), where hypothyroidism that has not been treated for a long time, that can occur during the aging process. Hypothyroidism is the most common thyroid disorder in America and one of the most frequent endocrine conditions worldwide. This is the one that has low thyroid gland function.

Fatigue, both mental and physical, is the characteristic of hypothyroid condition.

Thyroid Deficiency symptoms:

- Wake up with no energy
- Dry skin and thinning hair
- Constipation

- Problems with allergies
- Difficulty losing weight
- Feels cold even if the weather is warm
- High fatigue, exhausted feeling but not related to cholesterol, not responsive to diet, and not related to normal stress or amount of work or exercise
- Foggy brain and can't think fast
- Lethargic
- Anxiety, nervous, or panic attacks
- Voice is low
- Too much acne and some eczema
- Teeth marks at the edge of the tongue
- Swollen ankles and feet (water retention)
- Slow heart rate
- Face and palms are yellow
- Premenopausal and menopause symptoms are marked
- Abnormal menstrual period
- Diabetes, rheumatoid arthritis, or other autoimmune disorder
- Brittle nails
- Tremor of the hands and loss of balance for no reason
- Puffy face and bags under the eyes

Reverse T3

Most of the T4 is converted to T3 by our bodies by the peripheral tissues, the liver, and the kidneys. This is the pro-hormone for the T3, which is the one that is released to the blood stream. There is another product from T4 called reverse T3 (rT3). This has very low biological activity in the body. Due to abnormal metabolism or the aging process, there is more rT3 than T3. So due to this, the person can experience hypothyroidism symptoms. This is called Wilson's disease in which there is too much rT3 and not enough free T3 available for the cell to use.

The thyroid gland or cells do not shrink with age. The size can be normal but the external environment or toxins can influence the function and can cause disruption of the making of the thyroid hormone.

In *borderline thyroid disease*, we can also find:

- Adrenal insufficiency
- Protein malnutrition
- Loss of muscle mass
- Low level of vitamin B or folic acid
- Decrease of NK (natural killer) cells

In the case of hypothyroidism, we cannot assume that it occurs only during aging. This can be caused by other conditions, so finding the cause is always the goal in Integrative Medicine practice.

Thyroid hormone works synergistically with other hormones such as HGH, cortisol, and melatonin. I would recommend my patients without insomnia problems also take melatonin in the evening on a daily basis. Melatonin helps keeps us in good immune balance thus helping us to prevent cancer.

You can start with 1 mg/day at the age of forty and increase it by 1 mg every decade until 6 mg/day when you reach about seventy to eighty years old.

Progesterone

My favorite hormone is progesterone, and it is called the "protective hormone." In early 1990 the late Dr. John Lee, MD author of *Natural Progesterone*, brought this to public attention. He made the natural progesterone available in a jar where men and women can just purchase it over the counter. It has about 1 ½–3 percent progesterone made out of yam extract.

Many people get tested through saliva. Nurse practitioners were taught by Dr. Lee not to wait for conventional medical doctors to help them test the blood, so they tested the saliva. During this period many women appreciated these findings, and I was one of them.

Progesterone's benefits:

- Reduces the risk of ovarian and uterine cancer

- Helps with premenstrual cramps
- Helps migraine syndrome
- Improves osteoporosis
- Helps to balance cortisol
- Protects against negative side effects of excess estrogen hormone
- It is an anticatabolic hormone, protecting our bodies from destruction of cortisol (the stress hormone)
- Anti-stress, calming effect in men and women. Helps insomniacs.
- Progesterone is the direct production of "pregnenolone" (the mother hormone) using enzymes made in the mitochondrial cell of the ovaries, adrenal cortex, and other tissues.
- It produces testosterone.
- Women make more than men, and it peaks during midcycle.
- Barely detectable after menopause
- Improves mood and acts as an antidepressant
- Improves thyroid function
- Helps blood clotting
- Improves sexual libido for both men and women
- It is a neurosteroid and protects against brain cell damage
- Improves mitochondrial function thus improves energy production
- Improves vascular tone
- Improves immune system

Now you know why this is my favorite hormone among the others. Bio-identical progesterone is available and approved by many health insurance companies.

The Big Pharmaceutical progesterone is manufactured using a small amount of soy as a preservative so it can last longer than six months. It is good for people who can tolerate soy because it is more likely to be covered by their insurance company because it is made by pharmaceutical companies.

The compounding pharmacy makes it without the preservative but it must be labeled with an expiration date of six months. It is best to take this in the evening due to the calming effect.

ESTROGEN

Women need this more than men, and it significantly reduces the aging process. This hormone is what people say is "confusing" to take. Estrogen participates in the menstrual cycle, and prepares the uterus for conception. This is the female hormone that makes our skin beautiful and also increases our fertility.

There are three forms of estrogen based on its active form:

1. Estradiol E2 is the most active form. It affects every cell in the female body. When this is low, women have hot flashes; night sweats, thinning skin, anthropic or thinning gray vaginal mucosal tissues, insomnia, poor concentration, osteoporosis, and fatigue.

2. Estrone E1. This is the methylated form of estradiol and it comes as 20HE, 2 hydroxyestrone synthesized in the liver. (This form is the good form of estrogen and protects us from cancer activities). The researchers found out that if women convert estradiol to 20H about 40 percent, they have less risk of developing breast cancer (Meilahn 1998).

    The 16 OHE and the 4 OHE are the ones that can promote proliferation or induce DNA damage. This ratio influences cancer activity. Ratio of 2 OHE to 16 OHE is safe when it is higher than 2.

3. Estriol E3 is the end product of Estradiol and it has the most effect on lubrication for women.

Commonly in Integrative Medicine practice, when a physician replaces these hormones, we can use Tri-Est where you replace all forms of estrogen, or replace it with Bi-Est only where Estrone is excluded.

I tend to use the latter one as we can safely ignore the E1, as the estradiol will also turn into Estrone. Keeping the ratio balanced is a safer and more stable replacement.

Estrogen has the most complex endocrine relationship with other hormones. It works closely with LH (luteinizing hormone), FSH (Follicle Stimulating Hormone) and Prolactin, adrenaline, serotonin, endorphin, and dopamine.

During menopause age (45–60) estrogen drops to a constant low level when we can't see progesterone. FSH and LH will increase. These markers can be used to determine when women go into the premenopausal period. This period can occur from five to ten years prior to the real menopause when women do not have their period for at least six months. During the menopause period some women experience bleeding again due to regulating these hormones, but this period is un-ovulatory and it has only a psychological effect to women. They might feel that the aging process is somehow delayed.

In my practice I try to explain to them that some of them are still in the premenopausal period while having severe symptoms that affect their daily living activities, and will experience menopause stage using progesterone, but they feel great after that. Most women understand that after a certain age they do not have ovulation, and it is best to balance the hormone rather than waiting until the menopause stage to supplement it.

Statistically, 4 percent of the population among women do not go through any premenopausal symptoms and do not require any balancing of their hormones. They still have declined hormone levels.

There is risk in estrogen supplementation although the benefit has been long established by our researchers.

The risk of estrogen replacement includes:

- Fluid retention, swelling of extremities
- Bloating sensation
- Agitation, hypersensitivity, mood swings
- Inflammation in the body
- Increase of free radical damage
- Acceleration of aging if it is too high
- Migraine headache

- Breast pain and swelling
- Vaginal bleeding
- Stimulating one's genes in hormone-dependent tissues (breast, uterus, ovaries, and prostate).

Decisions need to be made, therefore you can't do it by yourself, and you need a professional practitioner to figure out the way to proceed by doing a routine follow up.

Benefit of estrogen replacement

1. It promotes renewal of CNS (central nervous system) cells in the brain.
2. Promotes regulation of the immune system and expression of cytokines.
3. Regulates growth factor including the skin growth factors so it protects your skin from becoming thin.
4. Increases production of growth hormone.
5. Prevents osteoporosis (bone loss).
6. Helps control the autoimmune process.
7. Prevents aging symptoms (a low level will accelerate aging).
8. Prevents cognitive and memory impairment.
9. Reduces risk of Alzheimer's (protects the brain from neurotoxins and oxidative damage), promotes neurogenesis.

AROMATIZATION

The process when the enzyme aromatase converts androgenic hormones to female hormones. Aging men and women can have low steroid hormones not produced by their aging organs. The older man, who gains more body fat than muscles, has more estrogen than testosterone. They aromatize more androstenedione and testosterone to estrogen. In this population, men increase the risk of having prostate cancer.

In a younger man, too much estrogen is not good. Aromatization can happen at any age especially those young men who use testosterone for muscle training purposes.

Due to estrogen increase, men can grow breasts and develop gynecomastia. This condition is irreversible and might need surgical intervention to remove them. Breast cancer can happen in men as well. I certainly would highly recommend a supervised steroid hormone replacement and not use the hormones sold in the black market.

In my practice, estrogen is barely used unless it is absolutely necessary, especially in aging men. For women if estrogen is appropriately prescribed and monitored, it gives them their youthful look back because it will also lower their biological age and helps to prevent sagging breasts and maintain healthy aging.

TESTOSTERONE

Anti-aging hormone also is referred as to the sex hormone. It helps both sexes in libido and sexual performance.
Benefits of Testosterone:

- Increases muscle mass and strength
- Helps balance estrogen and other female sex hormones
- Improves energy
- Lifts the mood
- Increases muscle tone
- Helps night sweats

ANDROPAUSE

This is the term for men that have declining testosterone due to aging. The onset is five to ten years slower than women. Most men have the andropause stage at the age of sixty or seventy.

Low Testosterone Symptoms

- Low energy, easily fatigue, weak
- Flabbiness of muscles
- Decreased muscle tone
- More abdominal fat

- Depression
- Low sexual libido, lost sexual interest in the opposite sex
- Decreases body hair
- No aggressive drive
- Night sweats

Normal Plasma level For Aging Men

Some of the range is not adjusted to healthy aging, and in my practice, patients responded to:

- Age 20–40 men is 600–1200 ng/dl
- Age 40–60 men is 500–700 ng/dl
- Age 60–80 men is 400–600 ng/dl

I routinely check the free Testosterone. I would like to see a free testosterone of >20–26 pg/ml.

For aging women:

- Age > 40 is 60–70 ng/dl I adjust it if they complain of having more facial hair, or hirsutism, which can be the effect of testosterone in women. It causes baldness in men called male pattern baldness, or alopecia.

The negative effect of testosterone replacement in women is low, but for men it increases risk of prostate cancer. Therefore we have to keep it in an acceptable range and optimal symptoms. Many European doctors have reported that testosterone does not increase risk or trigger prostate cancer. Lately they have reported using testosterone to treat prostate cancer. I would be very careful of a strong family history of prostate cancer for one whose PSA went up to > 4 ng/ml. Although PSA is not the best measurement for prostate cancer, I would still check this marker in all male patients.

I have encouraged my father who is now eighty-eight years old to keep using testosterone, and his PSA has always been lower than 1 ng/ml. He benefits from using this male hormone for over thirty years. Occasionally, I alternate it with secretagogues based on his results and his subjective complaints.

DHT (Di Hydro Testsosterone)

DHT is an excess conversion of testosterone into this dihydrotestosterone by 5 alpha reductase that is found in the prostate and also in the skin. This increase in DHT is associated with BPH, or benign prostatic hypertrophy, and an increased risk of cancer.

SHBG (Sex Hormone-Binding Globulin)

This increases during aging. This SHBG is testosterone that binds in the protein and will make the free testosterone unavailable to the receptors.

Higher SHBG can give low testosterone syndrome. Researchers found that restoring testosterone level could prolong health by prevention of heart disease or cancer.

Benefit of Testosterone

- Lessens fatigue
- Enhances sexual libido in men and women
- Improves muscle mass, tone, and strength
- Improves energy for men and women
- Increases youthful feeling and appearance

Bio-identical hormones

- I use only bio-identical hormones as much as possible before prescribing the others.
- I only replace hormones that are low in level.
- Follow-up laboratory results are very important to check the maintenance dose.

Typically there are three types of hormones in BHRT (Bio-Identical Hormone Replacement Therapy): progesterone, estrogen, and androgens. We can combine or prescribe single elements. BHRT is made of natural hormones, and because it has no patents or special monopoly right now, big pharma has less initial interest. Lately they are making progesterone, and it is called Prometrium with a small amount of soy as a preservative.

In my opinion this is a better solution when replacing hormones, but if one cannot tolerate this then I try any kind—even synthetic ones—that help the patients. Hormones are a sensitive issue when we first introduce them to our system. When patients have been on synthetic hormones for a long time and they get used to it, and then we change to this form, they feel different and afraid of the transition.

HORMONE TESTING

Before we start with replacement, we need to know the level so we can replace appropriately.

You need to have your hormone level tested.

TESTING:

- Blood level
- Dry urine testing/ DUTCH
- 24-hour urine
- Saliva
- Hairs

All of these levels can be used to gage hormone levels. Since the hormone is affected by biorhythm and they work synergistically with one another to create the neuroendocrine system, the physician who practices hormone replacement therapy has their own decision as to which test to use.

The most convenient test is of course the dry urine testing called DUTCH (dry urine test comprehensive hormone). However this test is not covered by insurance yet. The most common tests done by medical doctors are plasma levels or urine levels. A saliva test would cover both the free and total levels of hormones. It is commonly used, especially by those who are not able to get access to the blood due to poor venipuncture or small veins.

Balancing Hormones without Hormone

Some people are hypersensitive in taking hormones replacement even though it is a bio-identical hormone. We can help to balance their hormones by using some herbal remedies or nutraceuticals. These nutraceuticals work on the endocrine system, improving insulin mechanism and also modulating cortisol.

Exercise (aerobic and weight bearing on the big muscles) such as quadriceps, biceps, and back about fifteen to twenty minutes per day would help stimulate endogenous growth hormone release and helps to improve your essential fatty acid such as Omega 3 (EPA and DHA).

Fasting or calorie restriction was shown also to promote Growth hormone release. I encourage my patients and family to be on two weeks fasting with only one meal and Taking good replacement supplements for every three to four months. This helps us to clear the Phase 2 detoxification pathway.

Supplementation with amino acid stags can also improve the hormone secretion, especially when Secretagouges are taken on an empty stomach to get the best absorption though the stomach directly without going through the small intestine.

Some of these endocrine-nutraceuticals are

- Ascorbic Palmitate C
- E-Tocopherol 200–400 IU/day
- Co-enzyme Q-10 (Quinone)
- Alpha Lipoic Acid
- Magnesium 500–1000 mg/day
- Vanadium
- Chromium poly-nicotinate 200–400 mcg/day
- 7 Keto–DHEA 25–100 mg/day

- Melatonin 3–6 mg/day
- Pregnenolone 20–30 mg/day
- Phosphatidyl Serine 100–200 mg/day
- Poly peptide in Secretagogues such as Meditropin 2–3 pouches /day
- 5 HTP (Hydroxy Tryptophan)
- Adrenal Glandular 1.5–2.5 mg/day
- Thyroid Glandular
- Thyroxin 1000–1500 mg/day
- Bovine testicular glandular 15–30mg/day
- SAMe (200–400 mg/day
- B Complex
- Pantothenic acid 500 mg/day
- Methylcobalamine 1–3mg/day
- Folic acid or Methyl Folate
- DIM (Di-indol methane)
- Indole 3 Carbinol (I3C) 400–800 mg/day
- Saw palmetto 300–400 mg/day
- Plant sterols (Beta sitosterol)
- Isoflavones 100–200 mg/day
- Genestein 100–200 mg/day
- Lignans in flaxseeds 1–2 tablespoons /day
- Cinnamon for regulating insulin
- Wild yam root (Dioscorea)
- Licorice
- Garlic/ Kyolic
- L-arginine 10–30 gram/day
- L-lysine 1500–2000 mg/day
- Amino acid stack
- Leptin as Leptica AF
- HGH 1–1.5 IU 5–7 days/week every 4th month.

The list continues with many herbals in the list, among those are:

- Asian Ginseng (Panax), Siberian, Wisconsin, and many kinds of these approximately 100–200 mg/day. Some

people are sensitive to ginseng; it can be very "warming" and cause acne, but when it works, it also helps with energy.
- Velvet deer horn/antlers
- Ashwagandha
- Dong Quay
- Black Cohosh (Cimifuga Racemosa), Rimifimin

****

We thank Thee, God, for extra things
You send along our way
Both when our days are sunny bright
And when our skies are gray.

The little planned surprises dropped
From Thy great, loving hand,
Life unexpected showers on
A parched and desert land.

Just why you do these extra things
Our finite minds don't know;
It must be you delight in them
Because you love us so!

—Alice H Mortenson

Pillar VI

CELL REGENERATION

This pillar varies from several angles depending of the patient's condition during the aging period.
Some don't even need to explore this Pillar # 6, but at this stage in my practice, I find that the more education that is given about healthy aging, the more these pillars can be minimized.

This pillar includes:

1. Select your Integrative Medicine practitioner/doctor and work with your doctor. The doctor needs to oversee your healthy aging program.
2. Getting adequate hydration, take enough drinking water every day.
3. Replenish Electrolytes.
4. Check and boost your immune system.
5. Revitalize brain function.
6. Maintain homeostasis (sleep enough).
7. Maintain reserves (iodine, other minerals).
8. Recheck status at a minimum annually.
9. Cut unnecessary supplements and replenishing with what you need.
10. Check your status of bone, PAPS, and other necessary testing for plaques etc.
11. Avoid toxic environments.
12. Check bio-markers.
13. Personalizing your nutraceuticals.
14. Reveal information and share knowledge with your doctor, as not all doctors know everything.
15. Don't be afraid to integrate any pharmaceutical when it needs to be done and benefits your healthy aging.

Why do you need a medical doctor or doctor of osteopathy or naturopathic doctor? They need to properly prescribe alternative medications. Sometimes things happen, and you can have an infection that requires an antibiotic or antivirals. All hormones are regulated by prescriptions including human growth hormone and bio-identical hormones. There are more injectable vitamins and anti-angiogenesis for cancer that might need prescriptions. In fact, some of the good ones are not available over the counter.

Many of the esoteric nutritional companies only work with physicians because it requires knowledge to put together what seems to be our mother's prescriptions. Garlic, turmeric, echinacea, and cinnamon that you find in your kitchen for dietary use may not be concentrated enough to be used for its medicinal effect. One example is tea-polyphenols from green tea extract. This has no caffeine, and when it is concentrated and taken for only the polyphenol properties, each tablet is 650 mg that should be taken three times/day is equivalent to twenty cups of drinkable good green tea, three times/day (sixty cups/day). It is not possible for anyone to take this much good anticancer tea phenol in a regular tea drink.

One has to take forty carrots day to replace one 5000 mg of Beta-carotene capsule. One gram of fiber is equal to ten heads of lettuce, and we need 20–30 grams as minimum fiber/day. Can you imagine how much cabbage you would have to eat? It is more cost effective to take a nutraceutical than to eat that much produce.

One 500 mg capsule of malic acid and 150 mg of magnesium are equal to three apples. You need about 1500–3000 mg of malic acid for fibromyalgia and 800–1500 mg of magnesium/day. If you have to eat thirty apples a day that would be about $15/day and you could not tolerate it, whereas the capsule of that much nutriceutical will only cost you $1 per day.

There are many other examples that diet alone is not enough to guarantee your health. However we can give you some recipes or lists of food that you can select. The purpose is to avoid nightshade food for arthritis due to the arachidonic acid. Some people over do their cooking with olive oil and not realizing that it can tip off the ratios of Omega 3 to Omega 6. This also causes increased arachidonic acid that can cause joints to ache and pain without arthritis.

Many people are advised by their conventional physician not to worry about their diet and use of refined sugar. This is wrong as sugar can surely enhance the growth of active cancer cell as well once that is released to the blood stream.

PILLAR VII
EARLY DETECTION OF DISEASE

EARLY DETECTION

When you are diagnosed with a certain condition, you probably have a certain kind of feeling that is very personal.

If the diagnosis is solid and the symptoms have been chronic you may be surprised to discover you have a serious condition such as cancer. All kinds of emotional thinking can flood your mind. Sometimes it is very hard to accept the diagnosis and you feel like it is a dream not reality.

If the diagnosis is confirmed by objective findings but it is a pre- condition situation such as " pre diabetic", you probably will ask, how can I reverse it? You will hope to change what ever is necessary so you don't have to have the real Diabetic condition requiring a serious prescription medication.

If the diagnosis is more a "propensity " for a specific condition in the future, rather than a full blown illness you may feel and say " I don't think I will go there ".

Now days, using a new technology, some labs can help us to detect objective findings telling us these situations where a doctor like me can confidently say:

"Look, we find this accumulation of lipoprotein in your blood tests, and also an inflammatory markers indicating that this can be active plaque which can also accumulate and cause a stroke or heart attack in the future".

What are you going to say?

You may not believe that this is going to happen? You may not be obese, you may eat normally three times a day. However you may not know that you are carrying a mutated gene that can be now tested and it is the lipoprotein genetic findings where you were born with this gene. Probably your eating a normal diet, a normal american life style, where everything is ready cooked, and available in the super market for us who do not have the time to cook due to their work schedule. Yet you may find you are very ill. This situation is a common situation found in my office.

For the past 10-15 years, many improvements in technology have been made to help us preventive integrative medical doctors to detect this kind of situation.

Many more tests are now available to help the true carrier such as polycystic kidney disease in the Jewish community.

All of this can be detected to see whether they are a carrier where there is a certain percentage of risk but never is going to be expressed. Tests can determine if they are dominant, that is they can see from the test that whether they actually have this illness but symptoms are not out yet. That diagnosis can be now confirmed by this kind of test way before the patients are suffering from the actual symptoms.

I spoke to some of my friends who are handling directly this kind of test. For example, Dr. Schandhl of American Metabolic Lab has explained to me what his finding of his brother when he was found to have elevated of PHI (Phosphor Hexo isomerize) and sure enough 5 years later, his brother develop prostate cancer. He also mentioned about his sister who later on develop also cancer and she was found to have a positive finding years before.

I also conversed with doctors in several labs and I was impressed to find out that they can help me with difficult diagnoses when every thing else seems to be uncertain.

I did not have this luxury 30 years ago. I still remember that I had to spend almost US $ 20,000 just to look for the cause of a stroke in a 30 year old active healthy male who had a stroke. That was 35 years ago. Ten years later, my close friend who lives in France told me that I could check the c-RP (C reactive protein), which is one of the many other inflammatory and oxidative markers. Sure enough this CRP (C reactive protein) is usually elevated and it stir up the production of Fibrinogen and also the Apo B and Apo A lipoprotein which is the Plaque that either clog or break and travel to the brain and caused a stroke attack.

Now days there are many other markers which can be found as inflammatory indicators and Inflammation is one of the first markers in a cardio vascular disease work up.

The 1st – 6th pillars can be preventive measures. Each of them if done correctly, the patients will actually experience balanced health and likely lead to healthy aging,

With the early detection, we are able to uncover signs and let our patient know to be aware that they are carrying a certain risk and whether it is a moderate or severe risk of a condition

Some of these diseases are:

1. Cardio vascular events, stroke or heart attack
2. Pre diabetic
3. Syndrome X (Metabolic dysfunction, Hyperlipidemia with hyperglycemia and hypertension)
4. Insulin resistant
5. Leptin resistant
6. Pre Myocardial Infarction
7. Malignancy activities or cancer
8. Hormone imbalance
9. Menopausal stage
10. Prostatic activities in Enlarge prostate
11. Hypothyroid especially the subclinical one
12. Hyperthyroid
13. Low Immune system
14. Leaky Gut Syndrome
15. Imbalance essential fatty acid or deficiency
16. Memory impairment
17. Skin dryness
18. Osteoporosis And many more of course .

Many think they are just "getting older" and they deserve some of these symptoms, such as tiredness, fatique, shortness of breath with activities, pain in the joints or even headache and dizziness, repeated common cold, recurrent cancer sores or skin lesions that do not have any pain or itchiness. Constipation is also one of them or even the other opposite symptoms such as multiple diarrhea in a day and unexpected bloated stomach after eating something normal .

You probably heard this a lot too or may even have experienced some of these symptoms and have not thought of it as about any early detection of diseases.

Most people are used to taking over the counter non prescription medication for all of these symptoms. Unfortunately it is not the symptoms that you should treat but you should find the real cause, just like what I said in the beginning of this book. Don't only treat the symptoms but look for the causes.

Comprehensive test examinations in our office would cover automatically the basic early detections whether they come with symptoms or not.

1. Cardiovascular markers such as Lipid, Lipoprotein breakdown into Apo B and Apo A

2. Inflammatory markers (Fibrinogen, Myeloperoxidase, hs-CRP, and Lp-a)., the myocardial stress testings, etc.

3. Genetic evaluation on the Apo Lipoprotein, Platelets, Coagulation.

4. Metabolic assessment to include: insulin, FFA (free fatty Acid), Prediabetic markers, Vitamin D, B, Folate, Leptin, Adiponectin.

5. Essential minerals, Liver and kidney function, Protein,

6. Hormonal testings:

    Thyroid complete Panel (TSH, T4, Free T4, T3, Free T3)

    Adrenal function, Cortisol,

    Sexual hormone pathways : DHEA –So4, Pregnenolone, Progesterone, Estradiol, Estriol, Estrone, IgF-1, Testosterone and Free Testosterone.

Dry urine testing (DUTCH) is also a good test for people who do not like an invasive test.

Saliva specimen is also possible.

7. Basic Tumor markers:

   Lung CDT, CEA, CA125, C1-19, Ca1-15, PSA, Free PSA a

8. Essential Fatty Acid (3,6,9)

9. Oxidative measures : Iron or Ferritin with Compete Blood Count

All the Epigenetic factors are covered under many varieties of testing. Some are mentioned here :

1. DNA follicle "testing. This covers a basic:

   Leaky Gut for food allergy, Insufficiency of Vitamin, mineral, amino acid, essential fatty acid, fungus, bacterial and virus, radiation and additive allergy.

2. For detoxification we test for certain toxic elements.

   Essential minerals and detox elements

   Provocative agents often used to see a better results.

3. Immunology testing can be done by Genova blood testing. Or the above hair testing and common diagnostic lab.

4. "Pathway G Lab" genomic is offering a varieties of genetic test. They have the low risk test where we study the human DNA and understanding their propensity to help them understand better if they are prone to a certain epigenetic (diet/meal, activities/ exercise, nutrition, stress, hormonal).

5. Clifford Testing .

   This fits the early detection criteria for any chronic disease and inflammatory reaction. It is very useful for a dentist and patients who are interested in biological dentistry.

   The dental materials panel includes a wide range of materials divided into 36 categories used in treating your mouth such as fillings, crowns, implants, and orthodontics. The orthopedic panel covers surgical materials divided into 33 categories used to treat other parts of the body such as hips, elbows, and spines.

6. Early detection for Cancer :

   The fecal occult blood test (**FOBT**) is a lab test used to check stool samples for hidden (occult) blood. Occult blood in the stool may indicate colon cancer or polyps in the colon or rectum — though not all cancers or polyps bleed.

   The **Papanicolaou** test (abbreviated as Pap test, known earlier as Pap smear, cervical smear, or smear test) is a method of cervical screening used to detect potentially pre-cancerous and cancerous processes in the cervix (opening of the uterus or womb). This generally known as a PAPs Smear .

   The **HCG** (Human Chorionic Gonadotropin) Urine **test** was studied and introduced at American Metabolic Laboratories. This **test** is an important constituent of our**Cancer** Profile. We use this to find out if the cell are still multiplying. Part of our routine finding is to see if the patient is cancer free.

   Prostate-specific antigen, or PSA, is a protein produced by cells of the prostate gland. The PSA test measures the level of PSA in a man's blood. For this test, a blood sample is sent to a laboratory for analysis. The results are usually reported as nano grams of PSA per milliliter (mg/mL) of blood.

PSA (Prostatic Specific Antigen is often elevated in men with prostate cancer, and the PSA test was originally approved by the FDA in 1986 to monitor the progression of prostate cancer in men who had already been diagnosed with the disease.)

In 1994, the FDA approved the use of the PSA test in conjunction with a digital rectal exam (DRE) to test asymptomatic men for prostate cancer.

An alpha-fetoprotein (**AFP**) blood **test** checks of a pregnant woman can help see whether the baby may have such problems as spina bifida and anencephaly or chromosome disorder.

In men, non pregnant women, and children, AFP in the blood can mean that certain types of cancer-especially cancer of the testicles, ovaries, stomach,pancreas, or liver-are present. High levels of AFP may also be found in Hodgkin's disease, lymphoma, brain tumors, and renal cell cancer.

AFP (Alpha Fetal Protein)-L3 % (3rd electrophoretic Lentil Lectin %) = 10% is associated with a 7-fold increased risk of developing hepatic cellular carcinoma.

ONCO-Blot test which is testing for ENOX2, protein species resides inside the blood and is unique only to malignant cancer cells. These proteins serve as highly sensitive markers for early detection in both primary and recurrent cancer. These findings are based on research documented in Morre' and Morre', ECTO-NOX Proteins, Springer New York, 2013,

This test has the ability to identify 27 forms of cancer at their earliest possible development. That means it has the potential to detect cancer before other cancer screening tests on the market today.

A non invasive test or this is one of the Liquid Biopsy test or Blood biopsy.

Since this is an introductory book, I will not cover all tests. I will introduce other specific tests in future designated books for the condition mentioned in the book title.

Science will not stop developing. There will be much more testing that will allow us to know earlier before a real illness arises. This has been the case for the last 30 years.

Certainly **personalization** is the big key to anti-aging medicine using the integrative approach. From the initial test where personal history, objective findings and family medical history are all included in the initial decision to start the "detective " work of finding every illness in early stages.

We are very happy to see patients come back annually and find out if they are still having the luxury to enjoy their disease free status and maintain their healthy life.

- CTS (Chemo Sensitivity testing) can be utilized if cancer is confirmed to determine which drugs will be most effective for the patients. It is considered also as personalization therapy.

Genomic is a new common word in the medical diagnostic testings. Many tests ares now possible to be personalized. The National Cancer Institute describes this assay as a test that measures the number of tumor cells that are killed by the cancer drug. This test is done after the tumor cells are removed from the body . It is used to choose the best drug or multiple drugs for the cancer.

In some books that I have read and one of them is my reference book called " Are you sure ?" by Jenny Hrbacek, she states Genomic testing is not used enough by conventional doctors. Actually many Integrative doctors have used this test for many years and try not to use " one size fits all " cookie cutter treatments which is an old protocol from old schools.

Thank God that recently Integrative Medicine is part of the Specialty Physicians, and this way more and more conventional doctors can pay more attention to the new test in the field of early detection and prevention or even treatments. Especially in Integrative oncology where the diagnosis is almost like a death sentence due to the fear of the "one size fits all " treatment available in the world though conventional teaching. (They have nothing but to offer: Surgery, full dose Chemo therapy and radiation therapy).

More and more samples should be from Blood Biopsy. Labs in USA are more available now. We can reach many labs such as RGCC (Research Genetic Cancer Center) –www.rgccusa.com that has been established for many years to help us test for both the CTC and CST. They give us results that can detect the cancer cell and they will culture the cells to test it against the drugs.

Brain cancer is the exceptional because the cells can not be detected in the peripheral blood.

Obviously I love to recommend this test because the lab also test the biological or natural substance against the cancer cells .

OTHER "EARLY" DETECTIONS in Radiographic Technology:

(many of these tests can not detect early enough as you need to wait until the technology detect is at a certain stage), but most of these tests are the ones that are covered by an insurance or third party payor.

Commonly since many of this tests are going to be negative after patient's treatments, this is used to monitor the treatments and then we need to use the one that is such as CTC, CST, ENOX2, PHI etc.

With Radiation

1. Mammogram (sensitive to detect calcification findings)
2. CT Scan (Computed Tomography)

3. PET scan (Positron Emission Tomography)
4. All kind of X-rays for body and dental
5. DEXA (Dual X-ray absorptiometry (**DXA**) is the preferred technique for measuring **bone** mineral **density** absorption (BMD).**DXA** is relatively easy to perform and the amount of radiation exposure is low.

Early finding such as Osteopenia would help patient from going into osteoporosis.

6. **Spiral** computed tomography is a computed tomography technology involving movement in a helical pattern for the purpose of increasing resolution. Most modern hospitals currently use **spiral CT** scanners. **CT** beam types have included parallel beams, fan-beams, and cone-beams.

7. **Colonoscopy** is a test that allows your doctor to look at the inner lining of your large intestine (rectum and colon). He or she uses a thin, flexible tube called a colonoscopy to look at the colon. A **colonoscopy** helps find ulcers, colon polyps, tumors, and areas of inflammation or bleeding.

8. ColonSentry® is a convenient blood test that measures the expression of seven gene biomarkers (signatures) in the blood that are early warning signs of colon cancer.

9. Recently there has bee a scare because they are finding it difficult to cleanse the scopes completely.

10. Upper Gastrointestinal **Endoscopy**. Guide. An upper gastrointestinal (UGI) **endoscopy** is a procedure that allows your doctor to look at the inside lining of your esophagus, your stomach, and the first part of your small intestine (duodenum). A thin, flexible viewing tool called an **endoscope** (scope) is used.

11. **ERCP** is a **procedure** that enables your physician to examine the pancreatic and bile ducts. A bendable, lighted tube (endoscope) about the thickness of your index finger is placed through your mouth and into your stomach and first part of the small intestine (duodenum).

12. **Angiography** or arteriography is a medical imaging technique used to visualize the inside, or lumen, of blood vessels and organs of the body, with particular interest in the arteries, veins, and the heart chambers.

13. A **Holter monitor** is a continuous tape recording of a patient's EKG for 24 hours. Since it can be worn during the patient's regular daily activities, it helps the physician correlate symptoms of dizziness, palpitations (a sensation of fast or irregular heart rhythm) or black outs.

14. Medical Device 3-D scanner, this equipment is utilized for a quick testing in patients that usually are benefiting from an intra red or crystal treatment through an acupuncture meridian. This medical devised is approved by the FDA for a non invasive diagnostic and has been available for at least 30 years with fast improvement in its friendly user base and technology.

No radiation exposure test are: :

1. MRI, **Magnetic resonance imaging (MRI), nuclear magnetic resonance imaging (NMRI),** or **magnetic resonance tomography (MRT)** is a medical imaging technique used inradiology to image the anatomy and the physiological processes of the body in both health and disease. MRI scanners use strong magnetic fields, radio waves, and field gradients to form images of the body.

2. HALO Breast PAP test (A nipple aspirate device is a type of pump used to collect fluid from a woman's breast. A nipple

aspirate test can determine whether the fluid collected from the breast contains any abnormal cells.)

3. Thermogram, Thermography is a form of medical imaging capable of obtaining detailed infrared images of the human body.

4. Hair testing, A **hair test** can detect drug use for up to 12 prior months, but **accurate** results are typically limited to the past 90 days. In contrast, urine and blood-**tests** cannot **test** for use further back than a few days. This is why a lot of employers prefer the **hair follicle test**.

5. Epigenetic Hair follicle Analysis, this quick, uncomplicated and inexpensive process requires that we take 4-5 samples of hair from the nape of your neck and carry out testing and Using Epigenetic and breakthrough technology, with the root bulb attached.

    The information covers accumulated issues, current needs and even influences which are not yet detectable at a physical level. In other words before the cell weakness manifests into a period of incubation and potency that can then express as a symptom.

    It covers information for the person's Vitamins, Food Allergies, Viruses, Anti oxidant, Fatty Acid EFA, Minerals, Ciruses,Toxins, Microbiology and radiations.

6. Colonoscopy, is an exam used to detect changes or abnormalities in the large intestine (colon) and rectum. During a **colonoscopy**, a long, flexible tube (colonoscope) is inserted into the rectum. This procedure is invasive and has to be done by the Gastroenterologist specialist

7. Endoscopy, is to examine the esophagus (swallowing tube), stomach, and duodenum (first portion of small bowel) using

a thin, flexible tube called the upper**endoscope** through which the lining of the esophagus, stomach, and duodenum can be viewed.

8. An **ECG** is a simple, noninvasive procedure. Electrodes are placed on the skin of the chest and connected in a specific order to a machine that, when turned on, measures electrical activity all over the heart. Output usually appears on a long scroll of paper that displays a printed graph of activity on a computer screen.

9. Medical **ultrasound** (also known as **diagnostic sonography** or ultrasonography) is a **diagnostic** imaging technique based on the application of **ultrasound**. It is used to see internal body structures such as tendons, muscles, joints, vessels and internal organs.

10. Dark Filed Microscopy or Live Blood cell Analysis

The way to observe live blood cells under the microscope where it is magnified, viewed through this dark field microscope, magnified through a side way beam light, and you can see as it is projected onto a computer screen.. To see microorganism such as parasites, viruses and elements to evaluate immune system.

To end this Pillar VII I would like to share some of the symptoms that can lead us to early detection test .

- Unusual headache
- Unexplained dizziness
- Blurry vision that comes and goes or un usual
- Intractable pain
- Prolonged fever
- Fatigue and malaise
- Low energy despite a normal activities or long rest
- Skin color changes

- Yellow sclera
- Tinnitus
- Trouble swallowing
- Persistent cancer sore
- Unusual discharge
- Palpable abnormal nodules
- Itchiness
- Indigestions
- Pain in bowel movement and urination
- Blood in the stool or urine
- Shortness of breath
- Change in mood and personality
- Chronic cough
- Exposure to pesticide by accident
- Exposure to hazardous material
- Exposure to toxic material or water
- History of smoking cigarettes or as a long term secondary smokers
- Lives in a toxic environment
- Unhealed wound
- Depression
- Alcohol dependent
- Chronic viral infection (herpes)
- Overtime exposure to heats
- Strong history of cancer in the family
- Strong history of cardiovascular disease
- Suspect genetic disease (polycystic kidney or Parkinsons)
- Family history of cancer
- Poor diet
- Post chemo therapy
- Post radiation therapy
- Past history of recent cancer, not sure if you are cure .
- Suspect of unusual infectious exposure
- Recent visit of epidemic situation of infectious disease (hepatitis, typhoid, malaria)
- Unusual growth in body parts
- Premenopausal

- Pre andopausal
- Menopause
- Andropause
- PMS (Pre menstrual syndrome)
- Prolonged use of Birth control medication
- Prolonged use of any prescription medication
- Feeling unfit
- Yes,…not sure about anything and feeling un healthy
- Obesity
- Unexpected steady weight lost
- Never see a doctor for any check up for more than 3 years after age 25 (pre clinical stage of aging starts here)

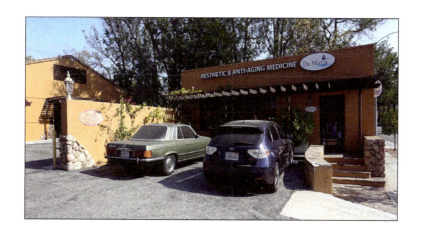

"God's Design"

Philosophers may reason why
But I wont take the time
I only know I'm here on earth
Because of God's design.
So I will just continue on
And do the best I can
And know that God will do the rest
Because He made the Plan.

—Ed Kane—

Chapter 8

The Practice and the Programs

THE PRACTICE

This place is my third location since I started my own private practice. It is a small but enough for my comprehensive practice in Integrative Medicine. In my practice, I incorporate all the pillars above, I review my formulas every six months or at the latest twelve months so I am not behind with the technology. This is what is best for my patients in term of supporting their healthy aging.

OUR OFFICE

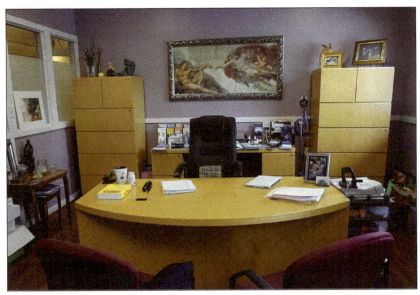

(Front office)

THE HYDROCOLONIC

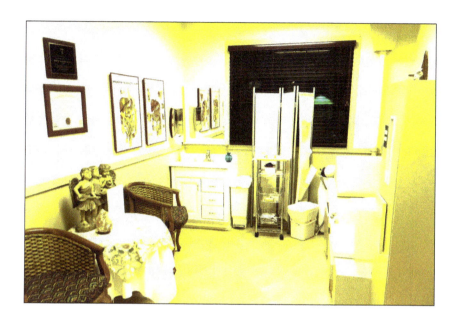

We offer oral and intravenous chelation together with the fractional intravenous push for any specific products or cocktails. All material comes from qualified certified and regulated compounding manufacturing companies and also pharmacies. Hyperbaric oxygen is one of the favorite besides of course the open system hydrocolonic.

I incorporate evaluation of the radioactivity exposure so this could be their first cleansing of the environment. Air and water are among the factors I discuss to educate my patients. In here we also incorporate biological dentistry.

HBOT (HYPERBARIC OXYGEN THERAPY)

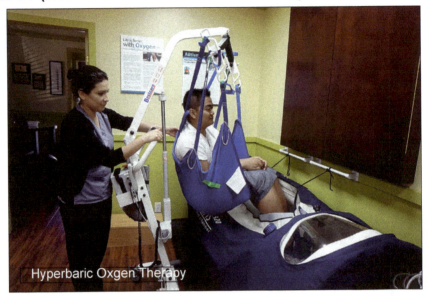

The Diet and Nutrition

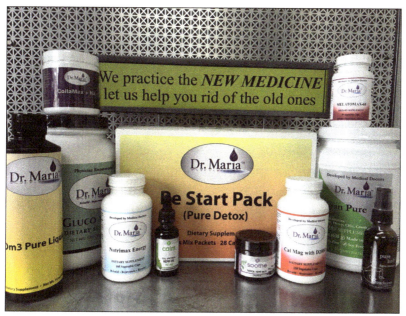

Compounding Supplements

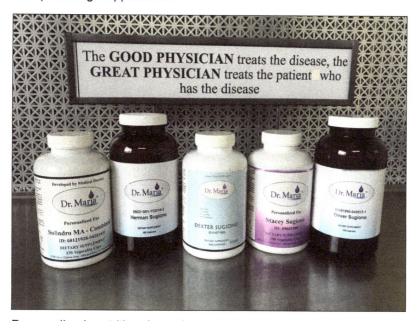

Personalized nutritional supplements based on one's blood, urine and hair testings

Hormone Balancing

I have incorporated the finest line of evaluation for diet and nutrition based on personalization of the patient and objective findings. That is the finest way to treat and measure results and will only improve the patient's trust. All decisions are based on the results of the diagnostic laboratories and their symptoms or goals. Safe weight reduction is also naturally done through evaluating their health condition first. We emphasize safe diet and weight. As I have mentioned above, if I have to prescribe a bio-identical hormone replacement or therapy, something that suits my patients, I use the most reliable sources. It must suit my patients, and of course this covers all ages from young adults to the centenarians. This is the most sensitive part of the human health system, yet it is often neglected due to misunderstanding about the negative or positive side effects and the benefit of these hormones.

Exercise:

This line is not foreign to me because of my primary training of physical medicine and rehabilitation at the UCLA residency program. I also personalize this to each individual and send them to appropriate trainer or therapist if need be.

The Practice and the Programs

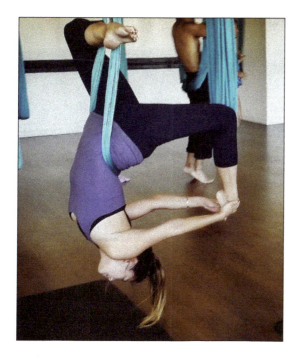

THE AIR YOGA -   **Stacey Sugiono -2015**

Stress Reduction

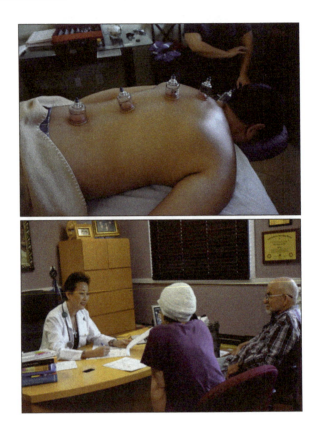

Since stress reduction is the factor than can tip over the rest of other pillars, I evaluate carefully by asking the patient questions. I try to help them to cut their medication by incorporating strong supplements and homeopathies to help them balance their mind and spirit. Hyperbaric oxygen therapy seems to help and the other pillars support this area, as well. Intravenous therapy also helps them. Currently, Ozone therapy is another option to up regulate organs that are under.

CELL REGENERATION

Major autohemotherpay using hyperbaric and high dose ozone is one of the option to boost cell regeneration.

This field is the fastest growing field. I make an effort to attend seminars in neuro-restoratology, stem cell and its fractions, and laboratorium to support this. Cell regeneration helps patients who seek looking young after feeling young and work with our qualified medical aesthetician to make their dream come true. I work closely with other medical doctors to accommodate what I don't have in the United States since the Europeans and Asians are far ahead of us.

OUR APPOINTMENT

We book patients according to their need but enough to do their initial evaluation and follow-up appointments with no double booking. Out staff are trained to exercise and understand all the pillars above. All patients are consulted with the aim of reaching their realistic goals. At the end of each consultation, they are also given their homeworks if any or the recommendation plan where this will be the step to reach their goals. The objective finding is always emphasized as a measurements. Testings are done to be our evaluation guide line and also the measurement of success forour program.

We use qualified up to date scientifically and high technology laboratories. We emphasize also the total integrative evaluation and also all possible reasonable genetic and DNA studies.

The personalized supplementation program in our practice seems to work very well to keep our patients happy and satisfied. Word of mouth is how we grow, and we appreciate the business that has been given from our patients and our colleagues or associate professionals.

Our patients are very special and they would feel special as well after walking out of our office.

****

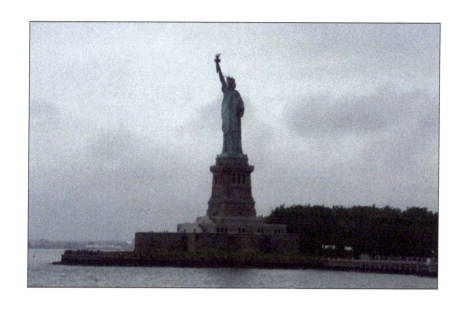

"Use Me Lord"

Lord, give me courage to be true
To you in all I say and do.
Give me your love to keep me sweet
To everyone I chance to meet.
Give me your power to keep me strong.
Grant me your presence all day long.
Give me the Faith that all amy see
How very real you are to me.
Give me wisdom to choose the best.
Help me perform each task with zest.
Give me vision to see your plan
Use me, Lord, wherever you can

Chapter 9

THE RESULTS AND TESTIMONIALS

I WAS PLEASANTLY SURPRISED TO FIND A HOLISTIC doctor who took Medicare insurance. The other doctors I had visited would not take any type of insurance. Then when I met Dr. Maria, I was surprised again that she took the time to find out all the medications but also all the vitamins as I am taking. Since then I have been introduced to new technologies that I was not aware of. Likewise I have been introduced to her very friendly and professional staff and even some of her family. I thank God for meeting Dr. Maria. I feel my health is in good hands now.

—**Don Bennett**
Los Angeles, CA
United States

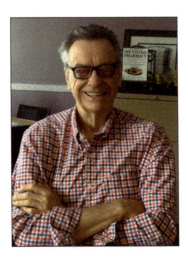

The Results and Testimonials

DR. MARIA HAS GIVEN ME MY LIFE BACK. HER BLOOD tests, for instance, go beyond most doctor's test. My internal medicine doctor did not understand how I received such thorough blood test to detect areas of my health that the conventional doctor would not normally be able to detect. My veins were infected, and the conventional doctors only knew one way : to send me to a cancer doctor who only wanted to dig deeper to find cancer with MRI, CT scans and blood tests that prove I had no cancer.

My vein was infected, and the conventional doctors only knew one way: to send me to a cancer doctor who only wanted to dig deeper to find cancer when MRI, CT scans, and blood tests proved I had no cancer. But Dr. Maria healed my vein through simple methods of antibiotic creams and calendula ointment (homeopathic).

—**Sharon "Shari" Mehr**
SM, CA
United States

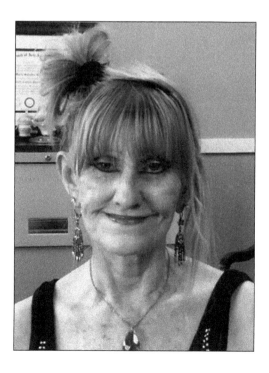

We are so grateful for Dr. Maria expansive wealth of knowledge of both Western and alternative medicines. Her kindness and commitment to educate her patients and to treat us with the most current and alternative modalities of healing has given us the opportunity to learn and experience safer, nontoxic ways to heal and maintain and improve our health.

—T. Mukai (92 years vibrant in 2015)
KT Mukai (daughter)
Los Angeles, CA
United States

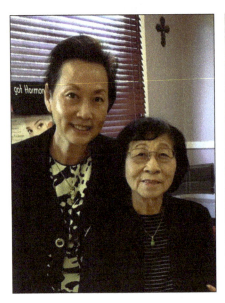
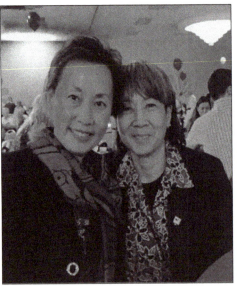

The Results and Testimonials

I USED TO TAKE DIFFERENT TYPES OF SUPPLEMENTS and multivitamins. They were good quality products, but I never really knew if I was taking the right kind and doses of supplements that my body needed. After my initial physical and consultation with Dr. Maria, I learned that my body was not as balanced as I had thought, and I had a higher inflammation, which I was not aware. My other primary care doctor could not detect this from normal routine blood test and could have resulted in serious health problems down the road if unattended.

Thanks to working with Dr. Maria for a couple years, it is great to see how balanced my hormones are and how great I feel now. It also gives me huge peace of mind to know that I am tracking and giving my body exactly what it needs to live harmoniously with ever-changing environments, seasons, and metamorphosis.

—**Cassie Sang**
Glendale, CA
United States

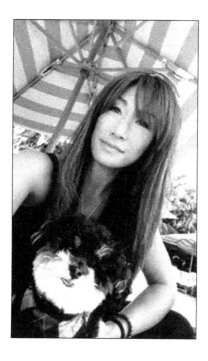

The No Coat Medicine

I HAD KNOWN DR. MARIA SULINDRO FOR OVER TEN years. Through my battle with post-polio and cancer, her methods and techniques have reduced my pain to almost zero. She has proved essential to my winning battle against cancer, and I owe her a large debt for providing answers and solutions to medical situations where traditional medicine has failed. I would recommend to any person to enlist her aid in anti-aging problems or any other medical situation that you may need resolved. As a person who has suffered lifelong with medical problems and visited many doctors, she tops them all. She also has a great social attitude, understanding the problems that you face, and provides a respect toward her patients that most doctors have forgotten or lost.

—Mark Kabacy
New Port Beach, CA
United States

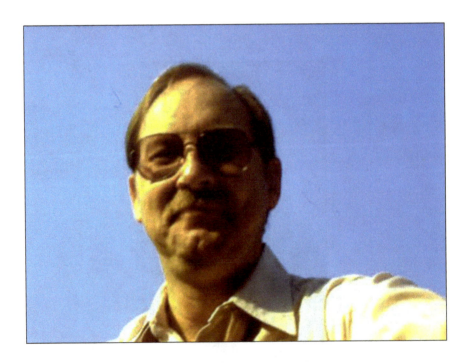

I AM A PRACTICING DENTIST IN WEST COVINA WHO has already been Dr. Maria's patients for twenty-five years. I was learning traditional dentistry and did not know much about alternative medicine and holistic medicine. When my thirty-one-year-old dental hygienist was so ill and could not walk, I knew she had mercury poisoning that I heard from Dr. Maria. She was healed in six months totally, and I am a holistic dentist now, doing what Dr. Maria also recommends. I take her personalized supplements and feel great , no tiredness and feeling full of energy and staying fit. No drugs. Thank God for Dr. Maria; she helps many of my patients.

**—Lillian Hon, 60
Pasadena, CA
United States**

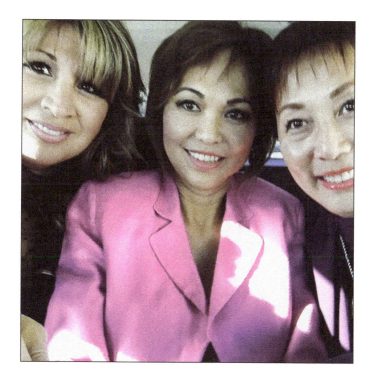

I AM FFTY-TWO YEARS OLD, AND DR. MARIA HAS BEEN my personal physician for more than a decade and, during the years, provided excellent care. Her personal attention to detail and genuine care for my health and life has given me the confidence to recommend not just my immediate family but dozens of others to visit her practice. She is a forward-thinking medical doctor. I have confidence putting my health care in her hands.

—**Eddie Stone**
North Carolina, CA
United States

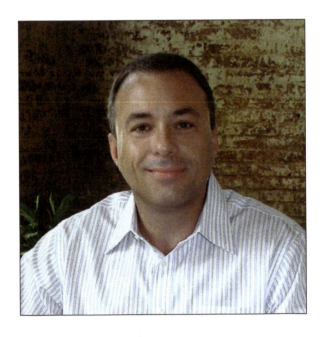

The Results and Testimonials

DR. MARIA HAS BEEN MY DOCTOR FOR MANY YEARS now, and has been a refreshing alternative to what I normally find in the medical profession. She looks at everything the world can offer a person to help manage, prevent, or cure, using both conservative and alternative methods that most medical doctors don't even know about.

If there is traditional medicine or alternative method out there that might help her clients, Dr Maria Looks into it, even if it was not what she was taught in medical school I have found a doctor who cares about me, and I am not afraid of getting older and being just a number anymore.

—**Kathryn Robbins**
Pasadena, CA
United States

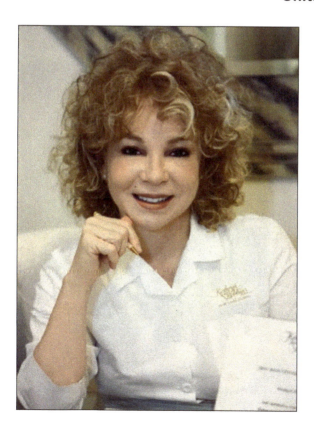

I HAVE BEEN UNDER DR. SULINDRO'S CARE FOR SIX months. My goal is to become healthier and less dependent on pharmaceuticals, which is becoming a reality. I've become accustomed to the supplements, B-12 injections, colonics, PT, and IVs. I have stopped taking statins, reduced high blood pressure medications, lost weight, and I am eating healthy and exercising regularly. I appreciate that Dr. Sulindro spends time discussing my progress and treatments, much of which is covered by Medicare insurance, thankfully. Her staff is always friendly and do their best to make you feel comfortable and welcomed.

—Stan Tsukahira
TC, CA
United States

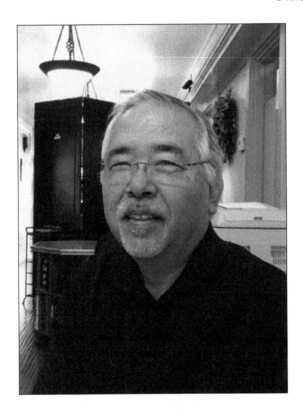

I WAS EXTREMELY LETHARGIC AND FEELING OLDER than all the senior citizens in my own family. I then started seeing Dr. Maria a couple years ago because my "traditional" doctors didn't have any expertise or training in Integrative Medicine. Dr. Maria helped me detoxify my body of heavy metals, balance my hormones, and identify nutrient deficiencies as well as food intolerances. Now with her personalized prescription plan for me (happy face), *I have never felt better*!

—**Susan Chan**
Rosemead, CA
United States

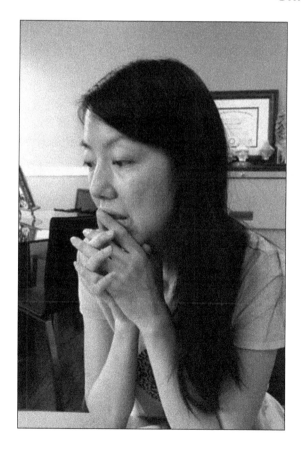

IN 1997, I WAS POISONED AND WITHIN THREE WEEKS was completely bald and the lymph nodes behind my ears were the size of a small eggs. I went to five doctors and had every test imaginable but their tests showed nothing abnormal. Everything came back OK. The doctors couldn't help me. So for fifteen years, I was on my own and tried everything possible to get well. During this time, through my own research, I discovered that I had fungus. My quest now was to find a doctor who dealt with fungus but couldn't find anyone to help me. I was so sick and desperate that I was considering going to Italy where there was a fungal specialist. Then in 2012, I found Dr. Maria. What a Godsend she was!

She gave me extensive blood work and other tests that the other doctors didn't know existed. These tests identified the fungus and the heavy metals (uranium, cadmium, and mercury, etc.), and I began treatment. Can you imagine my relief to finally find a doctor who could help me and who I could trust after suffering for fifteen years!

My primary physician had me on blood pressure prescription meds that had side effects. I told Dr. Maria that I didn't want to be on prescription drugs, and I knew I didn't need them. She put me on an enzyme and a supplement, and it worked beautifully and I got off the drug.

I am so thankful that I found Dr. Maria. She's experienced, intelligent, compassionate, and very effective. I have complete confidence in her and can relax knowing that I don't have to second-guess the doctors anymore.

—Maureen Kamph
Studio City, CA United States

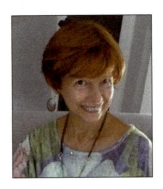

The Results and Testimonials

AS A PATIENT OF DR. MARIA FOR FOURTEEN YEARS, I have been on many programs, and I have lots of testimonials of what she has done for me. At the beginning, I wanted the best health money could buy and lose weight that was getting away from me. She worked hard with me, using personalized supplements for two and a half years and at the end of that time I was thirty pounds lighter, which called for a new wardrobe.

From time to time I had back problems, at which time she brought Dr. Wang in to help with my problems. Sometimes I don't listen to my body and lift things too heavy for me. In doing so, I experience lower back pain, and recently I had severe back pain that moved to the left side. Dr. Maria identified it immediately, and with four injections in the sore spots, I was once again helped by her knowledge of pain management. I think I learned what causes this problem, and where to go for relief.

—Arlene Townsend, 78
La Verne, CA
United States

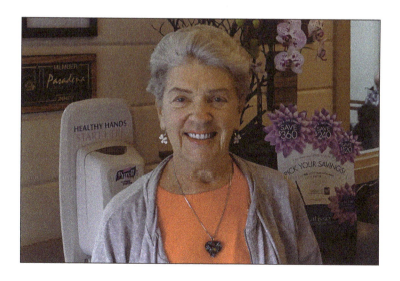

After being a patient of Dr. Maria for many years, I started to have problems going to the bathroom, so I called her office to make an appointment for a hydrocolonic. It was in January, and the holidays were over. I couldn't determine how or why this began to make me quite uncomfortable. The girl working with me was very competent and helped me a great deal. Afterward, the blockage cleared, and I felt normal once again.

In early August, I started to address the same symptoms as before with blockage in my urinary tract. With Dr. Maria's suggestion, I decided to start her program after a hydrocolonic and a blood test. I am taking supplements with her program to get me on the right track to further improvement while addressing prostate cancer.

—Roy Townsend, 78
La Verne, CA
United States

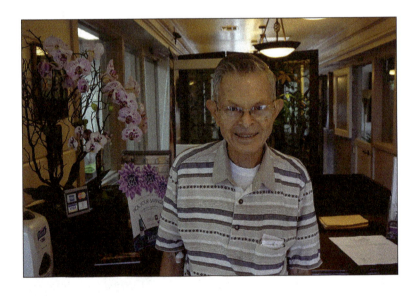

The Results and Testimonials

"SHE IS A HEALER WHO WITH HER HEART AND KNOWL-edge has helped thousands. She has introduced me to new ways and modalities of health and healing. I came to her with pain in my body, having already been seen many times by my former doctor. The secret to her guidance and medicine, I believe, is diversified guided treatments. She is extremely knowledgeable and will educate people in return. I have appreciated her treatments.

I love and thank you, Super Dr. Maria.

—Shayna Labeouf
California
United States

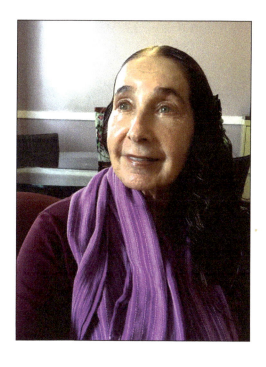

"I AM SO HAPPY TO HAVE DR. MARIA AS MY PRIMARY and only Doctor. She has made me feel so much better. I have been seeing her for approximately 3 years. She goes over and beyond the call of duty. She spends a lot of time evaluating my condition and communicating with me what I need to do to correct imbalances in my system, Thank God I was referred to her by a good friend. I will never see another Doctor. being in her care is like being in heaven."

—**Vicki Carlson**
Glendale, CA
United States

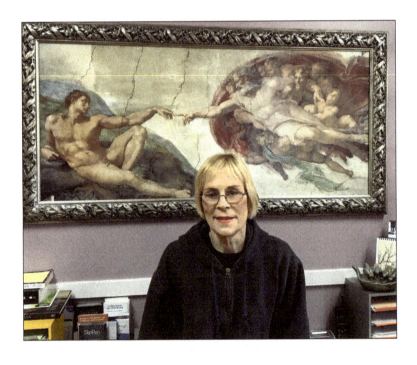

The Results and Testimonials

I HAVE KNOWN DR. MARIA FOR MANY YEARS . I CONsider she is my Anti-Aging Doctor. I am very happy to see results of her personalization that is made based on my blood test , urine or hair sample. She has been taking care of my health for preventive purpose. It is not for the look as people think but it is for internal health . Like Dr. Maria said to take care of internal health do we can be beautiful outside.

Thank you Dr.Maria for this advanced in medicine and I considered your program is very safe and helping people to stay away from the hospital. I want to grow old but still be very active and able to do what I want to do with my family and friends.

—**Dr.Hilly Gayatri DDS**
Kemang Jakarta- Indonesia

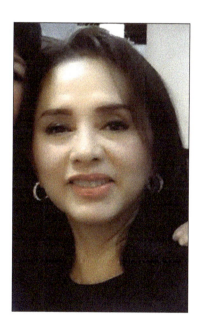

I HAVE TAKEN DR. MARIA PROGRAM FOR MANY YEARS, over than 20 years. Also I have taken health supplements for health care for many years.

I have always a good health and I want to extend this condition as long as possible. I began to take anti -aging supplements and program that Doctor Maria make special for me according to my blood test and many other tests. She told me not to take any extra of what I do not need. This is very important to know what not to eat and what you are lacking. Our body deteriorate when we grow older and of course if we take care and maintain the need to stay young , then you will feel young and good .My age is the same as Dr. maria's father. I always told Dr.Maria to give me the best as she always told me that she gave the best care to her father. I have good energy and I think the program works very well on me. Thank you Dr. Maria, for taking care of my health. People always think I look 10-15 years younger. I like to feel younger.

—Mooryati Soedibyo
Jakarta-Pusat, Indonesia

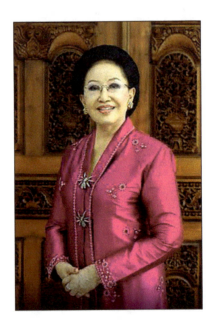

I HAVE BEEN DR. MARIA'S PATIENT FOR ALMOST 30 years . She has been taking a good care of my health using her Anti-Aging medicine program. Dr. Maria tries to not let me use drugs but using all organic and natural supplementation. I visited her beautiful office in Pasadena - California America , where she has all updated equipments and tests and she upgrades all the time. I feel greatful because I have a business to run and I go to work with full of energy, wake up with good attitude and work all day long without any problem or tiredness. I encourage people to do this type of care as this" New Medicine" does not ruin your health but improve and support your health. Our food and water and poluted if you are not careful, Dr.Maria takes her time to detoxify and allow our body to recharge . Her program also replenish what we are lacking. She also said that if necessary, we need to regenerate the weak cells.

But she does it without radiation or chemical but naturally. I do exercise, take care of good diet which is very hard because I love Indonesian foods. Instead of waiting for the serious illness to come,Dr. Maria check throuroughly and let my primary care doctor knows if I have any upcoming problem so I can reverse it. i just follow Dr.Maria's Integrative Anti-Aging program and it can maintain and sometimes improve my health to optimal stage . Dr. Maria change my program every 6 months, she does the compounding called Personalization. She makes it just for me and I always update my tests every year so she can make the best for me. I highly recomend this method of treatment to every one ".

—Abdul Latief
Jakarta - Indonesia

—**Abdul Latief**
Jakarta - Indonesia

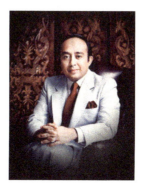

I HAVE BEEN A PATIENT OF DR. MARIA FOR SEVEN years. I have been following many of her programs. Among them are:

- Personalized supplements (she does not give unless is tested necessary)
- Hyperbaric oxygen chamber treatment, which has helped managed my everyday stress.
- B-cocktail injections
- Healthy vibrant hair
- Very athletic; I am seventy-four years young and still play tennis, ski, cycle, gym.
- Healthy memory/mind
- Gluten free now
- Healthy colon from hydrocolonic
- High energy and great eye function,
- No heart attack, nonsmoker, and no female problem or heat issues.

Thank you to Dr. Maria.

—**Elizabeth De Clifford**
Pasadena, CA
United States

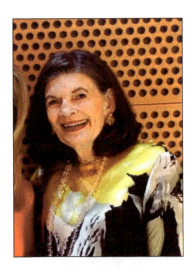

The Results and Testimonials

I HAVE BEEN SEEING DR. MARIA FOR SEVERAL YEARS and approve of her approach to medicine. I find that most doctors are brainwashed in medical school and are too quick to put you on drugs. With all the side effects caused by prescriptions, I am comfortable with a doctor, who is more aware, like Dr. Maria.

The program is very versatile and treats many conditions. The atmosphere in her clinic is pleasant, and her staff is lovely.

—Nina Cross
Covina, CA
United States

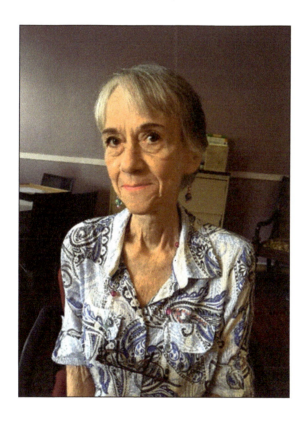

DR. MARIA HAS AN EXCELLENT INTEGRATIVE PROgram. Her knowledge is phenomenal and has helped me greatly. I also heard from other patients who have benefited from her care and personal attention. I hope more doctors would go into this field of medical care. I love the idea of not having to take medicine as a drug when supplements do such a tremendous job.

—**Johanna Rasmussen**
San Marino, CA
United States

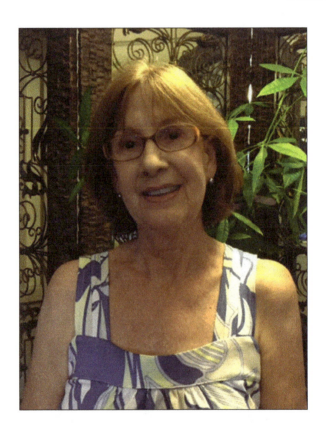

The Results and Testimonials

FIRST OF ALL I JUST WANT TO TELL ABOUT MY STORY. I had a small lump in my neck. I went to my doctor at Kaiser Permanente Hospital. The doctor told me that I had a lump in my neck, and I had cancer. I didn't know what to do. My friend used to buy Dr. Maria's medicine and told me to go to Dr. Maria. Bill is his name, and I have never gone back to my own doctor. Dr. Maria is the best doctor and tries the best she can. Now I am so happy to be her patient. Thank you, Doctor; you are the best.

—**Sina San**
Duarte CA
United States

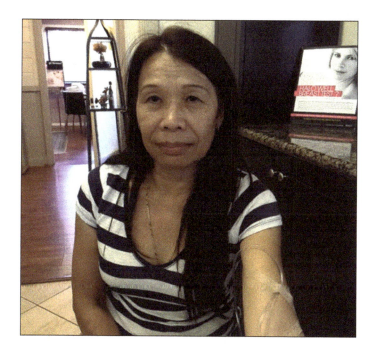

My experience of the hyperbaric oxygen treatment was that I was able to get relief from all of the pressure and weight of my mass that was obstructing my larynx and bronchial tubes, and I could breathe without an effort. I felt like I was floating and very exhilarated.

—Claire Boyer
N Hollywood, CA
United States

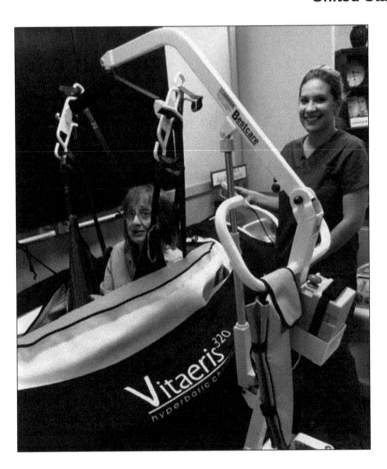

(Claire Boyer and Justine Gonzales MA)

The Results and Testimonials

I STARTED COMING ABOUT TWO WEEKS AGO, AND I can already feel an improvement. Everyone says my face looks brighter, and I feel stronger. I would highly recommend her care. Her staff is also the best.

—**Linda Ward**
Orange County, CA
United States

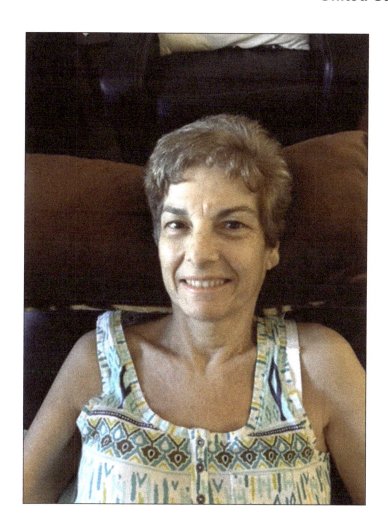

After the result of my urine laboratory workup, it was found that some heavy metals (mercury) and other metals were elevated. Dr. Maria recommended an IV chelation for detoxification. I also had tremors in my hand. Then she recommended an intravenous push of amino acids and other minerals. I have improvements in my tremor, and I am getting relieved.

—**Virgincita Alfonso**
Pasadena, CA
United States

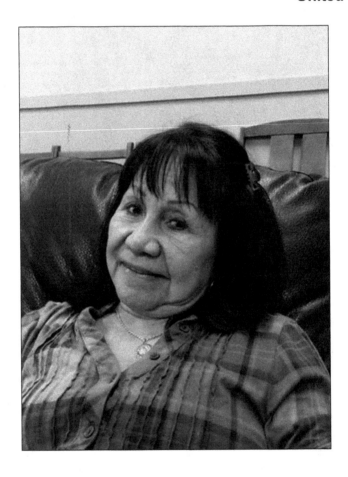

I HAD TRIED TRADITIONAL MEDICINE, BUT THERE DID not seem to be any good solutions to the myriads of physical issues I had. I found that Dr. Maria was very committed to "digging deeper" and trying to discover the root cause of my poor health. The practice incorporated many treatments that would help build up my body, rather than causing more problems—as I had experienced with taking drugs. I so appreciate Dr. Maria's expertise.

—**Linda Weigel**
Monrovia, CA
United States

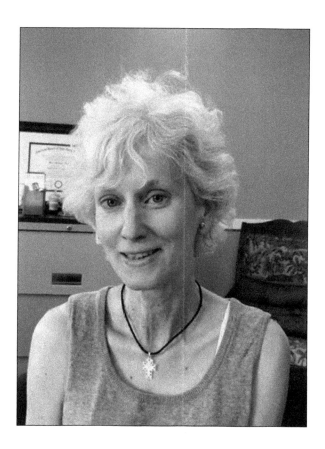

THE HYDRO COLONIC PROCEDURE IS A GREAT WAY TO keep your bowels clear. This can help to prevent any place for germs to build up. This is a simple procedure and is highly recommended as a preventive procedure for good health.

—**Robert Bum, Jr.**
Hesperia, CA
United States

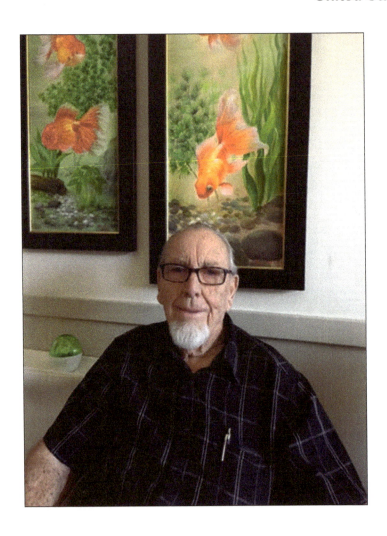

In 2010, I had a recommendation from a Chiropractor to see Dr. Maria for hormonal treatment. Several of her female patients had recommended her. On my first visit, Dr. Maria spent over an hour talking with me and getting a thorough picture of my history, and so forth. In a week or so, I had a blood test result, and from the results, she suggested supplements and hormones to balance my body system properly. She has a philosophy of using natural bio-identical hormones, which I agreed with. My energy improved, and I feel better after seeing her this past five years. One thing to note: when I follow the prescribed routine of supplements I have a properly balanced body system.

—**Valerie Wilding**
Pasadena, CA
United States

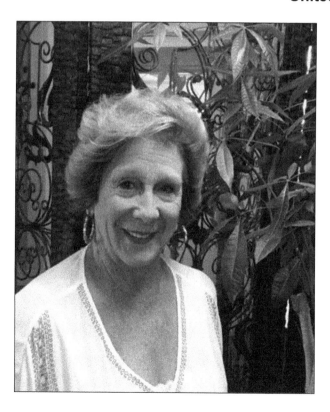

DR. MARIA'S DETOXIFICATION PROGRAM CHANGED my life! Before I did her program, I was constantly constipated and relied on the frequent use of a laxative (Dulcolax) for a time span of twenty years. After hearing this, she advised me to do a monthly hydrocolonic regimen and increase my intake of magnesium and probiotics. Now, my bowel movements are regular; I rarely experience constipation and feel healthier than ever before. With the clearance of my constipation, I have lost of a total of twenty pounds since starting her program two years ago.

**Marsha Hardy, 25
Temple City, CA
United States**

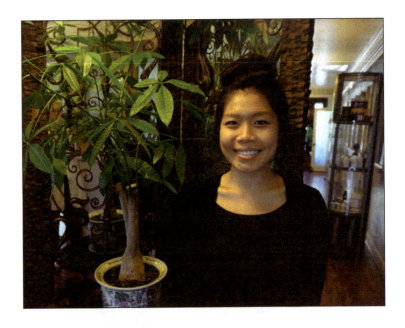

The Results and Testimonials

I HAVE BEEN A PATIENT OF DR. MARIA FOR THE PAST four years. She has helped me to rebalance my hormones and my health. Dr. Maria's approach to Integrative Medicine is the wave of the future, and she brings it to you now. I highly recommend Dr. Maria. She takes her time with her patients and is a caring, lovely woman. Do yourself and your well-being a favor and schedule a consultation.

**—Neva M. Smith
Burbank, CA
United States**

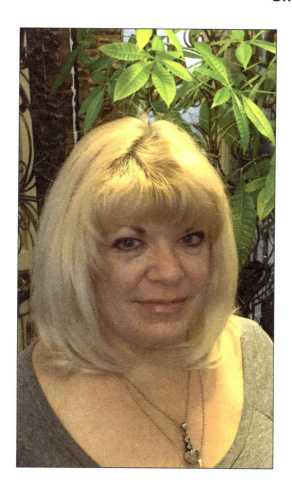

I HAVE BEEN A PATIENT OF DR. MARIA FOR EIGHT years. Most important is her practice of having blood test of the patient, dictating what my needs are in respect to specific vitamins and minerals and making for a more correct diagnostic analysis. This, I believe has helped me in taking what I need through the personalized powders without fillers, gluten, calories, and so forth versus taking so many vitamins in pill form daily.

She is very good in what she does, which is completely different than the typical practitioners. She also spends more time with you, and that is superior service compared to the fifteen minutes or so of the typical doctor visit (rush them in and rush them out) to generate volume dollars.

—Richard Berklite, 84
San Marino, CA
United States

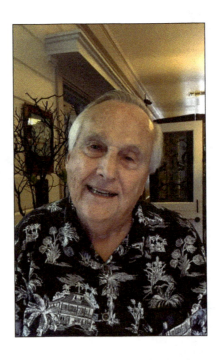

FEELING GOOD FEELS GREAT, AND FEELING BAD FEELS miserable. I am basically above average in living a healthy lifestyle and very in tune to my body. If I went to a standard doctor and said, "Something feels off," I would be asked very generic questions and leave without a confident resolve. This has never been the case with Dr. Maria. She knows the questions to ask to peel away the layers to find the underlying issue. A few thorough blood test—and not just the standard panel 20—and results are revealed. That's where my work comes in. If you put in the time, you get results, not over night, but in time. A change of diet a daily supplementation and adjust my bio-identical hormones, and voila! I am feeling better and repaired. Feeling good feels great!

—Carly Michaels
Delmar, CA
United States

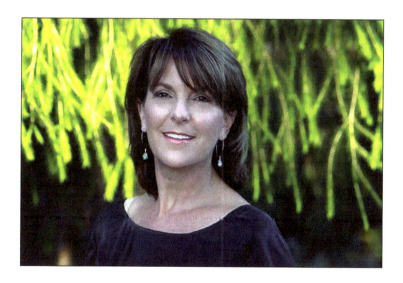

The No Coat Medicine

As we come to the end of this first book, I am reminded of a true story my friend Don tells me that illustrates a lot of what I have been trying to say in this book. It is about his brother Leonard. His older brother was a hardworking man, the beloved father of four boys and two girls. At the age of fifty-two, he had a heart attack.

Don went to visit his brother Leonard in the hospital. When Don arrived, his brother was in his hospital bed drinking coffee and eating chocolates that his loving but misguided friends had brought him.

Don immediately knew that is not wise and said, "Leonard, you can't be eating all that sugar and drinking coffee. You just had a heart attack." Leonard said, "Really? Why not?" Before Don could answer, the nurse walked in, and Leonard said "Let's ask the nurse." So Leonard asked the nurse "Is it okay for me to be eating these chocolates and drinking coffee?" She replied, "It's ok." "See?" Leonard says to his brother Don, "it's okay."

One year later, Leonard, after helping the Cub Scouts all day, had a big spaghetti dinner prepared by his friends. Then he had a second heart attack and died. He had a back-to-work order in his shirt pocket issued by the doctors at Kaiser. He was fifty-three.

Over twenty-five hundred years ago, *Hippocrates said, "Let food be thy medicine and medicine thy food."*

A little later, the great Apostle Paul wrote to the church at Galatia, *"Whatsoever a man sows that shall he also reap."* It is your choice, my friends.

"Choice"
Our live are songs;
God writes the words
And we set them
To music at pleasure
And the song frows glad,
Or sweet or sad,
As we choose
To fashion the measure.

-ella wheeler wilcox-

Doctors Contact and Information

Maria Sulindro-Ma, MD, ABAAM

Dr. Maria
Aesthetic and Anti-Aging Medicine

Integrative Medicine
Physical Medicine and Rehabilitation
EMG and Neuro-diagnostic Study

890 S. Arroyo Parkway
Pasadena, CA, United States
626 403 9000
626 236 5577 (fax)
www.MariaMD.com
email: askdrmaria@gmail.com
askDrMaria@MariaMD.com

Servicing women and men using Complementary methods:

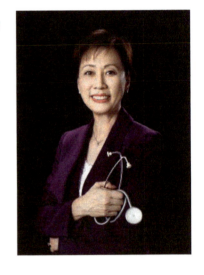

- Personalized metabolic therapy and weight management.
- Bio-identical hormone (compounded)
- Detoxification (all kinds)
- Hydro-colonic- open system
- Micro nutrition IntraVenous
- Hyperbaric Oxygen
- Cryosurgery
- Medical aesthetic rejuvenation, facial & permanent Make up

- Pain management, Prolotherapy, Joint Injections
- Hyperbaric Ozone, Major Auto Hemotherapy & Minor
- Polychromatic Ultra violet with LED and Multilights.
- Aesthetic : Skin Pen, PRP(Platelet rich plasma), Fillers
- Lipo Sage for fat reduction
- Memory testing
- Epigenetic hair Testing
- New Amsterdam Genetic Testing
- Personalized Nutrition based on your blood, urine & hair test.

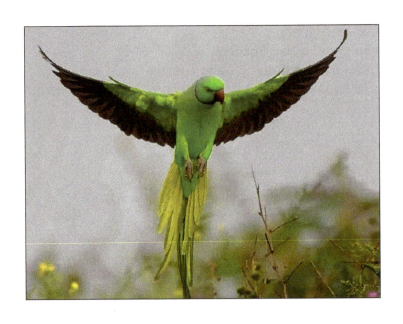

" Teach us, Lord, to serve thee as thou deserves:t:
To give and not count the cost;
To fight and not to heed the wounds;
To toil and not to seek for rest;
To labor and not to ask for any reward
Save that of knowing that we do thy will "

-St. Ignatius of Loyola-

Resources

MEDICAL ORGANIZATIONS

AAAAM (American Academy of Anti-Aging Medicine)
www.Worldhealth.net
www.A4M.com
1510 West Montana Street
Chicago, IL 60614
773–528–1000, 561–997–0112

AAEM (THE AMERICAN ACADEMY OF ENVIRONMENT MEDICINE)
www.aaemonline.org
316–864–5500
They offer education for physicians who are interested in the cause-and-effect relationship between environment and ill health.

ACAM (American College for Advancement in Medicine)
www.ACAM.org
380 Ice Center Lane, Suite C
Bozeman, MT 59718
1.800.LEAD OUT toll free; 888–439–6891
406.587.2451 fax
info@acam.org

AMERICAN ASSOCIATION OF INTEGRATIVE MEDICINE
www.aaimedicine.com
2750 East Sunshine
Springfield, MO 65804
417–881–9995

AMERICAN ASSOCIATION OF NATUROPATHIC PHYSICIANS
www.naturopathic.org
601 Valley Street, Suite 105
Seattle, WA 98109
206–298–0126

AMERICAN ASSOCIATION OF ORIENTAL MEDICINE
www.aaom.org
433 Front Street
Catasauqua, PA 18032
610–266–1433

ALTERNATIVE CANCER DOCTORS AND CLINICS
www.whale.to/cancer/doctors.html

AMERICAN HOLISTIC MEDICAL ASSOCIATION
www.holisticmedicine.org
6728 McLean Village Drive.
McLean, VA 22101–8729
703–556–8729

AMERICAN METABOLIC LABORATORIES
1818 Sheridan Streets
Hollywood, Fl 33020
www.americanmetaboliclaboratories.net
954-929-4814

AMERICAN OSTEOPATHIC ASSOCIATION
www.am-osteo-assn.org
142 East Ontario Street
Chicago, IL 60611
800–621–1773

BEST ANSWER FOR CANCER FOUNDATION
www.bestanswerforcancer.org
8127 Mesa, B-206, #243
Austin, Texas 78759
512–342–8181

ONCOLOGY ASSOCIATION OF NATUROPATH PHYSICIANS (ONCANP)
www.oncanp.org

NATIONAL CENTER OF HOMEOPATHY
www.nationalcenterforhomeopahty.org

CANCER CONTROL SOCIETY
www.cancercontrolsociety.com
2043 N. Berendo St.
Los Angeles, CA 90027
Phone: 323–663–7801 Fax: 323–663–7757

CANHELP, Inc.
www.canhelp.com
PO BOX 1678
Livingston, NJ 07039
800–364–2341

CENTER FOR ADVANCEMENT IN CANCER EDUCATION
www.beatcancer.org
130 Almshouse Rd suite 107 a
Richboro, PA 18954
888–551–2223

FOUNDATION FOR ALTERNATIVE AND INTEGRATIVE MEDICINE (FAIM)
www.nfam.org
PO Box 2860
Loveland, CO 80539

INTERNATIONAL ORGANIZATION OF INTEGRATIVE CANCER PHYSICIANS (IOICP)
www.ioicp.com
8127 Mesa, B-206, #243
Austin, Texas 78759
512-342-8181
Formerly known as the International Organization of IPT/IPTLD Physicians (IOIP), it was established in 2006

BIOLOGICAL DENTISTRY ORGANIZATIONS

HUGGIN AS APPLIED HEALING
www.hugginsappliedhealing.com
5082 List Drive
Colorado Springs, CO 80919
866-948-4638

INTERNATIONAL ACADEMY OF ORAL MEDICINE AND TOXICOLOGY (IAOMT)
www.iaomt.org
8297 ChampionsGate Blvd, #193
ChampionsGate, FL 33896
863-420-6373

TALK INTERNATIONAL
www.talkinternational.com
310-208-1158
888-708-2525

RESEARCH ORGANIZATIONS

AMERICAN SOCIETY ON AGING
www.asaging.org
833 Market Street, suite 511
San Francisco, CA 84103-182
415-974-9600

Resources

**CENTER FOR RESEARCH AND EDUCATION IN AGING
UNIVERSITY OF CALIFORNIA BERKELEY**
www.crea.berkeley.edu
401 Barker Hall, UC Berkeley
Berkeley, CA 94720-3202

**HUFFINGTON CENTER ON AGING
BAYLOR COLLEGE OF MEDICINE**
www.healthandage.net
One Baylor Plaza, M320
Houston, TX 77030
713-798-5804

NATIONAL INSTITUTE OF AGING
www.nia.nih.gov
31 Center Drive, MSC 2292
Building 31, Room 5C27
Bethesda, MD 20892
301-496-1752

LABORATORIES

AAL REFERENCE LABORATORIES
www.aalrl.com
1715 East Wilshire suite 715
Santa Ana, CA 92705
800-522-2621

AERON CLINICAL LABORATORY
www.aeron.com
1933 Davis Street, Suite 310
San Leandro, CA 94577
800-631-7900

AMERICAN METABOLIC LABORATORIES INC
www.americanmetaboliclaboratories.net
1818 Sheridan Street
Hollywood, FL 33020
953–939–4814

BIOFOCUS TESTS
Berghauser Str 295
45659 Recklinghausen
Germany
www.Biofocus.De
+49-2361-3000-130

CELLSEARCH
Janssen Diagnostic LLC
700 US Highway Route 202 South
Raritan, NJ 08869 USA
1-877-837-4339

EXACT SCIENCES LABS
www.cologuardtest.com
844–870–8870

CLIFFORD CONSULTING AND RESEARCH
www.ccrlab.com
4775 Centennial Blvd #112
Colorado Springs, CO 80919
719–550–0008

EXACT SCIENCES LABS
www.cologuardtest.com
844-870-8870

Resources

GENOVA LAB
www.gdx.net
63 Zillicoa Street
Asheville, NC 28801
United States

HEALTH DIAGNOSTIC LABORATORIES
www.hdlabinc.com
737 N. 5th Street, Suite 103
(Entrance is on Jackson Street)
Richmond, VA 23219
877–4HDLABS (443–5227)
804–343–2718
800–522–4762
828–253–0621

HEALTH DIAGNOSTIC AND RESEARCH INSTITUTE (HDRI)
www.hdri-usa.com
540 Bordentown Ave-Ste. 2300
South Amboy, NJ 08879
732–721–1234

INNOVATIVE LABS INC.
www.innovativelabsny.com
85 Commerce Dr.
Hauppauge, NY 11788
631–434–7514

LAB CORP OF AMERICA
www.labcorp.com
358 South Main Street
Burlington, NC 27215
336–584–5171

NEURO SCIENCE LAB
www.neuroscience.com
373 280th St.
Osceola, WI 54020
888–342–7272
877–282–0306

ONCIMMUNE LLC.
www.oncimmune.com
8960 Commerce drive, Building #6
De Soto, Kansas 66018
888–583–9030

ONCOblot Labs
1201 Cumberland Ave, Suite B
West Lafayette,, IN 47906
972-510-7773
www.oncoblotlabs.com

QUEST DIAGNOSTICS
www.questdiagnostics.com
One Malcolm Avenue
Teterboro, NJ 07608
800–222–0446

SPECTRACELL LABORATORIES, INC
Micronutrient testing
10401 Town Park Frive
Houston, Texas 77072
1-800-227-5227
www.Spectracell.com

RESEACRH GENETIC CANCER CENTER
RGCC, USA LLC
3015 Main Street
Rowlett, Texas 75088
214-299-9449

RED DROP TK TEST
En Garde Labs
97 Mountain Way Drive
Orem, Utah 84058
801-607-5096
www.en-garde.com

SINGULEX DIAGNOSTIC
www.singulex.com
1701 Harbor Bay Parkway, Suite 200
Alameda, CA 94502, United States
510–995–9000
888–995–6123

COMPOUNDING PHARMACIES

CENTRAL DRUGS COMPOUNDING PHARMACY
www.centraldrugsrx.com
520 W. La Habra Blvd.
La Habra, CA 90631
877–447–7077

COLLEGE PHARMACIES
www.collegepahrmacy.com
Colorado Spring, CO 80918
800–888–9358

INTERNATIONAL ASSOCIATION OF COMPOUNDING PHARMACIES (IACP)
www.iacprx.org
4638 Roverstone Blvd
Missouri City, TX 77459
281–933–8400

UNIVERSITY COMPOUNDING PHARMACY
www.ucprx.com
1875 Third Avenue
San Diego, Ca 92101
800–985–8065

I have no silver notes to turn
Into a lovely song,
But I can sit and listen
To a tune and hum along.

I cannot preach a sermon
To edify the year,
But I can say a little prayer
The Lord can always hear.

For though I do not preach or sing
Somehow I find a bit of God, …
… in every living thing.

—G Easley

THE NO COAT MEDICINE

Bibliography and References

ADVANCE GLYCOSYLATION end products in tissue and the biochemical basis of diabetic complications. Brownlee, M, A Cerami, et al. 1998. *The New England Journal of Medicine* 318:1315–21.

AGE BREAKERS. Borek, Carmia 2001. *Life Extension* (August):39–43.

AGING SUCCESSFULLY with complementary medicine. Aldridge, Susan 2001. Novartis Foundation for Gerontology (www.healthandage.com).

AGE RELATED CHANGES of Dopamine receptors in the rate hippocampus a light microscope auto radiology study. Amenta, F, F Mignini, A Ricci, et al. 2001. Mechanism of Aging and Development 122(16):2071–83.

A HYDRICYCHALCONE derived from CINNAMON function as a mimetic for insulin in 3T3-L1 adipocytes. *Journal of American College of Nutrition* 20(4);327–36.

AMERICAN CANCER SOCIETY 2002. Cancer Facts and Figures 2001. New York: American Cancer Society.

APPLE CIDER VINEGAR
Paul C Bragg, ND., PhD, *Health Science.*

ARE YOU SURE ? (CANCER FREE)
Jenny Hrbacek, RN, *New Voice* 2015.

ARE GONADAL STEROID HORMONES INVOLVED IN DISORDERS OF BRAIN AGING? Azcoitia, I, LL, Don Carlos, and LM Garcia Segura 2003. *Aging Cell* 2(1):31–37.

ASSESSING BENEFITS AND HARM OF HORMONE REPLACEMENT THERAPY: Clinical applications. Nelson HD 2002. *Journal of the American Medical Association* 288(7):882–4.

A WORD OF CAUTION: Can Growth Hormone Accelerate Aging? Bartke, A 2001. *Journal of Anti-Aging Medicine* 4(4):301–09.

BABESIA UPDATE 2009 ROUTINE AND ADVANCED TESTING OFTEN FAIL. Standard treatment does not cure. James Schaller, MD, Randal Blackwell. Hope Academic Press. 2000.

BIOLOGICAL THEORIES OF AGING. In *Endocrinology of Aging*. Kamel, Hosamk, Arshag Mooradian and Tanverr Mir.2000. Totowa, New Jersey: Humana Press.

BLOOD GLUTATHIONE decreases in chronic disease. Lang, CA, BJ Mills, W Mastropaolo, et al. 2000. *Journal of Laboratory and Clinical Medicine* 135:402–05.

CANCER IS FUNGUS, A revolution in Tumor Therapy, DR. T Simoncini 2007 lampiz Edizioni

CALORIC RESTRICTION IN NON MAMMALIAN MODELS. Gerhard, Glenn S. 2001. *Journal of Anti-Aging Medicine* 4(3):205013.

CHRONIC INFLAMMATION: The Epidemic Disease of Aging. Falcon, William. 2002. *Life Extension* (January):13–16.

CURCURMIN INHIBITS INTERLEUKIN 8 PRODUCTION AND ENHANCES INTERLEUKIN 8 RECEPTOR EXPRESSION ON THE CELL SURFACE: Impact on Human Pancreatic Carcinoma

Growth by Autocrine Regulation. Hidaka, H.T. Ishiko, et al. 2002. *Cancer* 95(6):1206–14.

DEHYDROEPIANDOSTERONE replacement in aging humans. Flynn, MA, D Weaver-Ostergolytz, et al. 1999. *The Journal of Clinical Endocrinology and Metabolism* 84(5):1527–3.

EFFECT OF DL-ALPHA LIPOIC ACID ON GLUTATHIONE METABOLIC ENZYMES in Aged Rats Arivazhagan, PK Ramanathan and C Panneselvam. 2001. *Experimental Gerontology* 37(1):81–87.

EFFECT OF A HOMEOPATHIC DRUG. CHELIDONIUM in Amelioration of p-DAB Induced Hepatocarcinogenesis in Mice. Biswas, SJ and AR Khud-Budksh 2002. *BMC Complementary and Alternative Medicine* 2(1):4–12.

EFFECTS OF HUMAN GROWTH HORMONE IN MEN OVER 60 YEARS OLD. Rudman, D, AG Feller, HS Nagraj, et al. 1990. *New England Journal of Medicine* 323:1–6.

EFFECT OF TAI CHI EXERCISE ON BALANCE FUNCTIONAL MOBILITY; and fear of falling among older women. Taggart, HM, 2002. *Applied Nursing Research* 15(4):235–42.

ENDOCRINE EFFECTS OF DIETARY RESTRICTION AND AGING; Mtlison, Julie A, GS Roth, et al. 2001. *Journal of Anti-Aging Medicine* 4(3):215–23.

EPIGENETIC—The death of the genetic theory of disease transmission. Joe D Wallach, BS, DMV, ND, Ma Lan, MD, MS Lac, Gerhard N Schrauzer, PhD, MS DACn,CNS, Select Books 2014.

ESTROGEN METABOLISM: a complex web. Liska, DJ, and LR Leupp, 2001. *Journal of the American Nutraceutical Association* 5(3):4–14.

EVERY HEART ATTACK IS PREVENTABLE Bartke.2001. Washington, DC: Lifeline Press.

FROM FATIGUE TO FANTASTIC Jacob Teitelbaum, MD. Avery 2001.
HEAL YOUR HIPS—How to prevent hip surgery and what to do if you need it. Robert Klapper, MD, Lynda Huey, John Wiley and Sons Inc.1999.

FUNCTIONAL MEDICINE ADJUNCTIVE SUPPORT FOR SYNDROME X. Functional Medicine clinical practice protocol. Lukaczer, Dan, 1998. Gig. Harbor. Washington: Health Comm International.

GLUTATHIONE: systemic protectant against oxidative and free radical damage. *Alternative Medicine Review* 2(3):155–76

HEALING THROUGH NUTRITION A natural approach to treating 50 common illness with diet and nutrients. Melvyn Werback, MD Author of Nutritional Influences of Illness. Harper Collins 1993

HUMAN SALIVA AS A DIAGNOSTIC SPECIMEN. *Journal of Nutrition* 131 (5):1621S-25S.

HOW TO STAY YOUNG AND LIVE LONGER. Maria Sulindro, Michael Lam. 2002 Academy of Anti-Aging Research, Inc.

HORMONAL CHAOS: The scientific and social origins of the environmental endocrine hypothesis. Krimsky; Sheldon. 2000. Baltimore, Maryland: John Hopkins University Press.

HYPOTHYROIDISM. The unsuspected illness. Barnes, Broda O, and L Galton 1976. New York: Harper and Row.

IMPROVING GENETIC EXPRESSION IN THE PREVENTIVE OF DISEASES OF AGING. Bland, Jeffrey S 1998. Gig Harbor, Washington: Health Comm International.

INSULIN SIGNALING. Bevan, P 2001. *Journal of Cell Science* 114(8):1429–30.

INFLUENCE OF DIETARY SUCROSE ON BIOLOGICAL AGING. McDonald, RB. 1995. *American Journal of Clinical Nutrition* 62(1):284S-92S.

INSULIN RESISTANCE: lifestyle and nutritional influences. Kelly, G. 2000. *Alternative Medicine Review* 5(2):109–32.

LEPTIN AND PRODUCTION. Catacane, VD, and MC Henson. 2002. *Seminar in Reproductive Medicine* 2(2):87–88.

LOW GLYCEMIC INDEX: Lent carbohydrates and physiological effects of altered food frequency. Jenkins, DJ, AL Jenkins, TM Wolever, V Vuksa, AV Rao, LU Thompson, and RG Josse, 1994. *American Journal of Clinical Nutrition* 59 (3rd Edition):706S-09S.

MASTERING THE ART OF SELF RENEWAL. Hudson, Frederic M. 1999. New York:MJF books.

MITOCHONDRIAL AGING, open questions. Beckman, KB and BN Ames 1998. *Annals of the New York Academy of Sciences* 854:118–27.

MICRO CURRENT PREVENT CANCER AND DELAY AGING. AMES, BN, 1998. *Toxicology Letters* 102–103:5–18.

OPTIMUM ENERGY FOR PEAK PERFORMANCE. Sylvia Poobalasingam, MD, Fusion Excel INT. 2007.

ORALLY ACTIVE INSULIN MIMICS. WHERE DO WE STAND? Balasubramayam, M and V Mohan, 2001. *Journal of Bioscience* 26(3): 368–90.

OXIDATIVE DAMAGE to mitochondrial DNA is inversely related to maximum life span in the heart and brain of mammals. Barja,

Gustavo and Asuncion Herreto 2000. *Journal of American Societies of Experimental Biology* 14:312–18.

PUSHING LIMITS OF THE HUMAN LIFE SPAN, Kolata, Gina 1999. *The New York Times* (March 9).

PROGESTERONE MODULATES THE EFFECTS OF ESTROGEN ON IGF-1 IN POST MENOPAUSAL WOMEN. *Growth Hormone and IGF Research* 8(4):1431–45.

PROSPECTS FOR HUMAN LONGEVITY. Olshanky. S Jay, Bruce A Carnes, and Aline Desesquelles. 2001. *Science* 291(23):1491–92

RADIATION: Unsafe at any dose. Mitchell, Teri, 2001. *Life Extension* (November):40–47.

RELATIONSHIP BETWEEN AGE, DEHYDROEPIANDOSTERONE SULPHATE AND PLASMA GLUCOSE IN HEALTHY MEN. Nihal. T, HA Morris, et al. 1999. *Age and Aging* 28:217–20.

REGULATION OF THE IMMUNE RESPONSE by Dehydroepiandosterone and Its Metabolites. Loria, RM, DA Padgett, and PN Huynh. 2996. *Journal of Endocrinology* 150 Supplement:S209–20.

SERUM URIC ACID AND CARDIOVASCULAR MORTALITY. Fang Jing and Michael H Alderman. *Journal of American Medical Association* 283–2404–10.

SLEEP AND MORTALITY. Kripke, DF. 2003. *Psychosomatic Medicine* 65(1):74.

SOY AND ITS ISOFLAVONES. Brynin, R. 2002. *Alternative Medicine Review* 7(4):317–27.

TREATMENT OF H. PYLORI INFECTED MICE WITH ANTIOXIDANT ASTAXANTHINE REDUCES GASTRIC

INFLAMMATION, BACTERIAL LOAD AND MODULATES CYTOKINE RELEASE BY SPLENOCYTES. Wadstrom, T and LP Andersen. 1999. *Immunology Letters* 70:185–89.

PROLONGING HEALTH J.E. Williams, O.M.D., Hampton Roads. 2003

MELATONIN, IMMUNE MODULATION AND AGING. Zhang, Z, PF Inserra, et al. 1997. *Autoimmunity* 26(1):43–53.

METABOLIC ABNORMAL in growth hormone deficient adults: II carbohydrate tolerance and lipid metabolism. Beshyah, SA. A Henderson, et al. 1994. *Endocrinology and Metabolism.* 1:173–80.

NATURAL HORMONE REPLACEMENT. Jonathan Wright and John Morgenthaler. 1997. Petaluma. California: Smart Publications.

NATURAL KILLER CELLS, viruses and cancer. Cerwenka, Adelheid, and Lewis L Lanier 2001. *Nature Reviews Immunology* I (October) 41–49.

NATURAL PROGESTERONE: The multiple roles of a remarkable hormone. Lee, John R. 1993. Sebastopol. California: BLL Publishing.

NEW DRUG TARGETS FOR DIABETIC TYPE 2 AND METABOLIC SYNDROME. Mooler, David E 2001. *Nature* 414:821–27.

NUTRITIONAL CONTROL OF AGING. Zimmerman, JA, V Malloy, R Krajcik, et al. 2003. *Experiment Gerontology* 38:47–52.

NUTRITIONAL SUPPLEMENTS professional edition. Lyle Mac William MSc, Fp—Northern Dimensions -2007

NUTRITION AND SUPPLEMENTS FOR PAIN MANAGEMENT. Maria Sulindro-Ma, Cherise L. Ivy,

Amber C Isenhart 2000. Integrative Pain Medicine. The science and practice of Complementary and alternative medicine in Pang Management-Springer.

Oxygen Free Radicals and Systemic Autoimmunity. Ahsan, A Ali and R Ali 2003. *Journal of Clinical and Experimental Immunology* 131(3).398–404.

TABLE of Worldwide Living Supercentenarians. 2001 *Journal of Anti Aging Medicine* 4(3):267–69.
Journal of Anti Aging Medicine 5(1):141.

TELOMERE State and Cell Affects. Blackburn, Elizabeth H.2000. *Nature* 408:53–56.

The Aging Brain; Normal and Abnormal Memory, Albert MS 1997. 1999. *Transaction of the Royal Society of London* 252 (1362):1703–09.

THE CHINESE HERBAL MEDICINE Metria medica. Bernky, Dan and Andrew Gamble 1986. Seattle: Eastland Press.

THE FOOD DOCTOR Healing foods for mind and body—Vicki Edgson Sipion and Ian Marber Sipion. Collins and Brown. 1999.

THE IMPACT OF GLUTATHIONE on Health and LONGEVITY. Lang, CA. 2001. *Journal of Anti-Aging Medicine* 4(2):137–45.

THE LIVER CLEANSING DIET. Cabot, Sandra 1996. Scottsdale, Arizona: SCB International.

THE MIRACLE OF ENZYME self-healing program—Hiromi Shinya,MD–qanita 2009.

THE CHINA STUDY T Colin Campbell, PhD and Thomas M Campbell II, Benbella 2006.

THE COMPLETE GUIDE TO ANTI-AGING NUTRIENTS
Hendler, Sheldon S. 1985. New York: Simon and Schuster.

THE GROWTH HORMONE SECRETAGOGUES counteracts glucocorticoid-induced decrease in bone formation of adult rats. Andersen, NB, K Malmlot, et al. 2001. *Growth Hormone and IGF Research* 11:266–72.

THE HEALTHY LIVING SPACE: 70 practical ways to detoxify the body and home. Levingston, Richard. 2001. Virginia: Hampton Roads Publishing Company.

THE HORMONE SOLUTION. Hertighe, Theirry. 2002. New York Harmony Books.

THE MALE MENOPAUSE–does it exist?. Goud, Duncan C, Richard Petty, and Howard S Jacobs. *British Medical Journal* 320(March):858–61.

THE NEW GLUCOSE REVOLUTION. Brand Miller, J, TM Wilever, K K Foster-Powel, et al. 1996. New York: Marlow and Company.

THE OKINAWAN PROGRAM Learn the secrets to healthy Longevity. Bradley J Wilcox, MD, D. Craig Wilcox, PhD, and Makoto Suzuki, MD–Three Rivers Press 2001.

THE ROLE OF CARBOHYDRATES in insulin resistance. Bessesen, Daniel H. 2001. *Journal of Nutrition* 131:2782S-86S.

THE SCHWARZBEIN PRINCIPLE II. Schwarzbein, Diana. 2002. Deerfield Beach, Florida; Health Communication.

USE OF ISCADOR. An extract of European mistletoe (*Viscum Album*), in cancer treatment: prospective nonrandomized and randomized matched-pair studies nested within a cohort study. *Alternative Therapies in Health and Medicine* 7(3):57–78.

UNWRITTEN KNOWLEDGE. Diamond, Jared 2001. *Nature* 410(March 29):521.

WHAT DO WE REALLY KNOW about the risks and benefits of growth hormone and IGF-1? Injections, secretagogues, and testing. *Townsend Letters for Doctors and Patients* (Dec):90–92.

Meet the Author

Maria Sulindro-Ma, MD ABAAM was born in Indonesia, a third generation Chinese. She is known as Dr. Maria and has been a practicing medical doctor in Pasadena, California for more than thirty years. She is a specialist in anti-aging Integrative Medicine.

Dr. Maria received her medical degree from the University of Indonesia in 1980. She completed her internship in neuro-psychiatry at Loma Linda University, California and completed her post-graduate residency in physical medicine and rehabilitation at UCLA in 1987. She is an active member and certified by the ACAM, ABPM, Chelation and Toxicology, Acupuncture and Herbology Medicine, A4M where she has served as oral board examiner for many years.

She was the founder of Academy of Anti-Aging Research for Physicians with accredited medical education. For her practice she incorporates oxidative medicine, hyperbaric oxygen therapy (HBOT), MAHT (Hyperbaric ozone Therapy) , Polychromatic light therapy, detoxification , homotoxicology, intravenous cocktail therapy with nutritions and also Nutritional personalization, prolotherapy, homeopathy, bio-identical hormone replacement, cell regeneration, and other supportive treatments. She is a frequent speaker in national and international medical conferences, public education and has written books. She pioneers the "Personalized Anti-Aging Nutritional Program" using objective findings. Her motto is "Internal beauty is the key to healthy aging."

For more information, visit **www.MariaMD.com**
or call her office at: **626–403–9000**
email: **askdrmaria@mariamd.com** or
askdrmaria@gmail.com

"Resolve"

Build on resolve, and not upon regret,
The structure of thy future.

Do not grope among the shadow of old sins,
But let thine own soul's light
Shine on the path of hope
And dissipate the darkness.

Waste no tears upon the blotted record of lost years,
but turn the leaf and smile, oh, smile,
To see the fair white pages that remain for thee.

Prate not of thy repentance, but believe the spark divine
dwells in thee; let it grow.

That which the up-reaching spirit can achieve
The grand and all creative forces know;

They will assist and strengthen as light
Lifts up the acorn to the oak trees height.

Thou hast but to resolve, and lo! God's whole great universe shall fortify thy soul.

—Ella W Wilcox

CPSIA information can be obtained
at www.ICGtesting.com
Printed in the USA
FSHW011034090619

9 781498 454650